HEALING THE AILING MEDICAL SYSTEM

Homeopathy Leads the Way

Ashok RajGuru

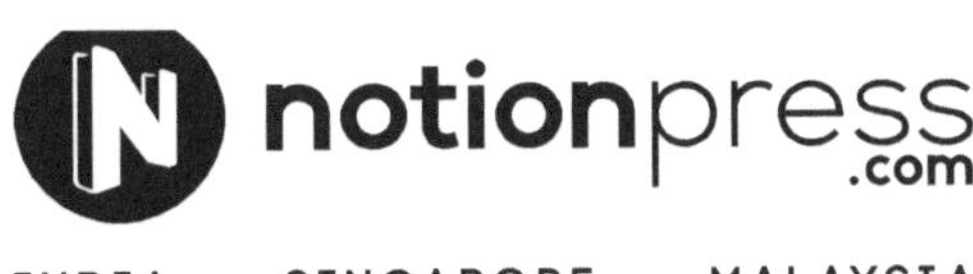

ISBN 979-8-89363-930-8

Dedication

To my wife Anjali, who has been my most profound inspiration &
support.

Ancient Sanskrit Proverb: सुभाषितम्

वैद्यराज नमस्तुभ्यं यमराजसहोदर।
यमस्तु हरति प्राणान् वैद्यो प्राणान् धनानि च॥

O Vaidya (Doctor), I bow to Thee
Brother of Yama (God of Death).
Yama seizeth one's life alone, whilst
Thou seizeth one's wealth as well.

Contents

CHAPTER 20 Care for the Elderly **169**

CHAPTER 21 Ars Moriendi: The Art of Dying **175**

Acknowledgements

"Appreciation is a wonderful thing. It makes what is excellent in others belong to us as well."

– Voltaire

The idea of creating this sourcebook was suggested by many who wished to find a single resource that collated information and references that they could refer to when faced with unfounded criticism or biased writing against homeopathy.

I wish to acknowledge my debt to all my teachers in the Art of Healing. It all began with Khurshed 'Bawa' Batliwala and Michael Fischman of The Art of Living Foundation who brought me to this Path.

I have been guided in this journey by Padma Bhushan Dr. David Frawley (a.k.a. Pandit Vamadeva Shastri), Padma Shri Vaidya Rajesh Kotecha, and Michael Reid-Kreuzer (later Buddhist Monk Losang Jinpa).

My deepest gratitude to my teachers at the British Institute of Homeopathy both in the United States and England, namely, Maria Bohle, Lynn Cremona, the Late Donna Earnest, Dr. Trevor Cook, and Sandra Burroughs – thank you for the thorough grounding you provided me in classical homeopathy.

I thank my clinical guides under whom I interned, Dr. Dinesh Chauhan of Mumbai and Dr. Subrata Kumar Banerjea of Allen College of Homeopathy, Kolkata.

Thanks to Dr. Rajan Sankaran and Grant Bentley for the insightful courses in my continuing education.

I am deeply indebted to Dr. Will Taylor, MD for teaching me anatomy, physiology, disease and pathology from the whole-person, homeopathic perspective instead of the reductionist and mechanistic approach taught in medical schools.

I have learnt a great deal from Dr. Rajesh Shah, whose book I had the privilege to edit, and from which I learnt so much that transformed my practice.

I thank Dr. Manish Bhatia, and Mr. Alan Schmukler of *Hpathy*, the popular and most widely read international homeopathy journal for their support and encouragement.

Thanks to Dr. Amarsinha Nikam and his son Dr. Manish Nikam for providing access to their hospital for evaluating the efficacy of homeopathy in a hospital setting.

I acknowledge my debt to my patients without whose trust and support I would have made no progress in my journey.

Pune, India.

– Ashok RajGuru
PhD, DHM, DIHom, BFRP
Instructor, Fellow & Member of the Board of Advisors
British Institute of Homeopathy International,
NJ, USA.
Website: https://ashokrajguru.com/
www.youtube.com/@WiserOwlsAcademy

Prologue

"The unequal distribution of power in contemporary society is reflected and reproduced in medical ideology."

– D. Flic

The Western medical system based on the current model has gone terribly wrong – and this book shows how we might go the right way again. In the future, healthcare system will hopefully put the needs of its most important stakeholder, the patient, first. The way forward is to integrate the wisdom of other systems of medicine and create a holistic approach which includes traditional medicine to Homeopathy - the true medicine of the future.

This sourcebook is a concise collection of carefully analysed data gathered during the course of my years of study, practice, and research. It will provide the reader with authentic sources of evidence of the efficacy of homeopathy and help practitioners of other systems of medicine to incorporate the methodology in their day-to-day practice after examining the evidence presented.

Currently, the medical establishment exercises influence not merely over medical matters but also over social, cultural, ideological, and economic spheres of life. This was particularly evident during the Covid-19 pandemic. This is a sort of medical hegemony of allopathy enforcing its dominance over a narrow bio-physical model of healthcare along with a vigorous suppression of alternative models of healing and cure, like homeopathy. This happens with the "corporatization" of personal and clinical medicine into a pharmaceutical industry-led, hospital-centred treatment. The financial might of the pharmaceutical industry is greater than the international armament industry. According to the

Stockholm International Peace Research Institute, the world's largest arms-producing and military services companies generated a revenue of US$ 597 billion in 2022 (SIPRI, 2022). Compare this with the sales of the pharmaceutical companies worldwide which amounted to a whopping US$ 1.48 trillion during the year 2022, which is two and a half times the global expenditure on armament (Statista, 2023). It is interesting to note that in the year 2023, the global market of homeopathic products was valued at just US$7.11 billion, or less than one half of one percent (0.50%) the value of the pharmaceutical companies' sales (Fact.MR, 2023).

The effects of this supremacy are all too obvious to miss. The primary structure of this hegemonic structure is based on the triad of the insurance industry, pharmaceutical industry, and the medical associations like the American Medical Association or the Indian Medical Association etc. Today, a large part of their revenue is generated by disease mongering, that is, convincing healthy people that they are sick and require medicines. This sort of disease-mongering has turned ordinary conditions like baldness, erectile dysfunction, restless leg syndrome, and a host of other conditions into medical problems. Every human condition is sought to be medicalized. There is no disagreement with the fact that medical journals have played a paramount role in terms of educating health professionals on this controversial phenomenon. Indeed, pharmaceutical companies sponsor diseases and promote them to prescribers and consumers (Moynihan, Heath, & Henry, 2002).

This domination and control are reflected in the recent complete exclusion of the subject of "family medical practice" from the Bachelor of Medicine and Bachelor of Surgery (MBBS) course curriculum in India. It is disappointing to note that the discipline of Family Medicine has been entirely excluded from the MBBS curriculum. The words such as 'Family Medicine', 'Family Physician', 'General Practitioners', and 'Family Practice' have not even been mentioned once in the entire 83 pages of the draft MBBS curriculum document. This is shocking because a family doctor is the patient's first contact in all health systems across the world. Further, this is not an inadvertent occurrence or a default situation. The Medical Council of India played a significant role in diminishing the role of family physicians in the Indian health system. Interestingly, family medicine has been recognized as a distinct specialty in India for several decades but has not been included in the undergraduate (MBBS) curriculum/training till date (Kumar, 2023).

As a matter of fact, the word "family doctor" has been gradually replaced with an impersonal and sterile term – "primary healthcare provider". The family doctor used to be the patient's best chance of getting individualized and personal care. But that does not fit into the corporatization of healthcare as it was an independent and private enterprise. Today, a doctor would unhesitatingly give a cortisone injection for tendinitis in the ankle, which is covered by health insurance and is the approved hospital protocol, rather than recommend a shoe insert that may just as well work. The alternative, holistic, whole-person oriented therapies too do not fit into the corporate structure and are therefore hounded out. That is why many home-based treatments, such as some geriatric care and cancer care, which though cost-effective and preferred by patients, are never encouraged. That is because current payment systems don't routinely cover this care (Shmerling, 2021).

It is in these circumstances that we must look beyond the current bio-physical model of health. Indeed, the role of modern medicine in surgery and emergency care cannot be denied, but its wider influence over our society must be reduced. We should also take note of the fact that according to data published on the US government website Consumer Financial Protection Bureau, a 2019 study (pre-Covid-19) found that 66.5% of all personal bankruptcies were tied to medical bills (consumerfinance.gov, 2023).

Today allopaths can actually play a key role in combating disease-mongering. But do they have a choice? What can they do? We shall look at how homeopathy promises to be a more universal, inexpensive, and effective form of cure, which can be incorporated in any clinical practice. It is truly the Medicine of the Future.

This book is neither propaganda for homeopathy not a monotheistic doctrine. It is an invitation to allopathic physicians, homeopaths, practitioners of other Healing Arts as well as laypersons to evaluate, adapt and incorporate principles that will improve their results in day-to-day practice. For the allopaths it will offer new insights to heal their patients, and some may well cross over to homeopathy. The homeopath will be inspired with greater confidence and conviction in the system because this book presents tremendous amount of data and evidence supporting homeopathy. The layperson will be able to make a fair evaluation and an informed choice in matters relating to their health and well-being. The healers from other disciplines will be able to draw inspiration and adapt practices to help their clients.

This sourcebook will promote a deeper, more meaningful understanding of the complex issues that surround life sciences in general and the Healing Arts in particular. It is my hope that eventually Homeopathy will bring medicine home – to heal the sick.

Introduction: Towards Wiser Healing

"The doctor of the future will give no medicine but will instruct his patients in the care of the human frame, in diet and in the cause and prevention of disease."

– Thomas Edison

The current western medical system is ailing. It seems to be governed by a "Deep State" run by the triad of the pharmaceutical industry, hospitals and insurance companies. This has deeply affected the wellbeing and health of the common man. Sadly, the attempts to heal this ailing system are largely political initiatives aimed at providing populist measures limited to insurance-based solutions like Medicare or Medicaid. It does not address the deeper malaise.

We live in a world where science and technology have greatly impacted our lives. Advancements in medical technology should have led to improved treatments for diseases and illnesses. Also, advances in mental health research should have better supported mental health. However, what we often find is that while treatments have advanced, healing has not. Once upon a time "bedside manner" was a physician's most potent medicine. Today, the medical system has degenerated into a technology driven industry to generate revenue. But beyond financial adjustment, authentic reform will have to come from reinstating ancient, intimate healing relationships between patient and doctor. Homeopathy is perhaps the only medical system that can provide the leading light to the path of affordable, personalised patient care.

The following anecdote will illustrate the suffering of the present-day common man (Stange, 2009).

A wealthy man once went from doctor to doctor to try to find a reason for his fatigue. Each doctor looked in depth at the organ in which she/he was an expert. Each did the latest diagnostic tests. Each prescribed the latest drugs and devices. And the patient, the person only got worse. He was in charge of his healthcare, he bought the best of each commodity, but in the end his fatigue remained, and he only felt lonelier and more isolated.

What the man experienced was treatment, but the outcome was quite the opposite of healing. Healing requires relationships – relationships which lead to trust, hope, and a sense of being known. But our healthcare system doesn't deliver healing anymore. It doesn't deliver relationships. Increasingly it delivers commodities that can be sold, bought, quantified, and incentivized. The wholistic outlook that caters to whole people, whole systems, whole communities—gets worse. While governments, health care systems, and individuals spend more and more on healthcare, they get less and less value.

The key idea in the passage quoted above is the need for wholistic healing and individualised care, and a closer, compassionate doctor-patient relationship. This can all be delivered by homeopathy at a fraction of the cost of the current medical system led by the triad mentioned earlier and improve care, recovery, and healing.

Here is another parable regaled by Dr. EW Berridge, MD in a medical journal of 1881 (Berridge, 1881).

In that dim, mystical, prehistoric epoch known as "Once upon a time," two knights, traveling in opposite directions through a forest, came simultaneously upon a shield suspended from the branch of a tree. Thereupon they stopped to examine it and began to discuss what it might mean. At length one of the knights remarked that it was made of gold, and the other replied that it was made of silver. They began to dispute about this, and presently came to blows.

Some hours afterward a third knight came up, and finding them both lying on the ground, wounded and unable to rise, inquired the cause. Having heard what had occurred, he informed them that they were both right in their respective assertions as to the composition of the shield, but that each was wrong in maintaining that he alone was right, for the shield had two different sides, one of gold and the other of silver. Whereupon the two combatants, the stranger having bound up their wounds and assisted them to rise and mount, rode away, each a sadder and a wiser knight.

What the anecdote informs us is that while individual points of view may be correct in a narrow way, they are invariably one-sided and therefore incomplete. The opposition to homeopathy and other complementary methods by the practitioners of allopathy reminds us of the anecdote of the two warring knights mentioned above. That is the root cause of the elusive "healing". It has been the experience of countless people that many well-intentioned actions sometimes have the unintended consequence of making things worse.

The need of our times is to develop a WISER outlook – the word WISER being an acronym for an outlook that is *W*hole-person oriented, *I*ntuitive, *S*imple, *E*ffective and *R*ational. Integration of healing practices from across the world that span many millennia of accumulated knowledge, experience and wisdom is the need of the hour.

A paradoxical payoff has been discovered in primary healthcare worldwide which is often missed by doctors. The paradox is that better whole-person and system outcomes are observed despite apparently poorer quality disease-specific care (Rao & Pilot, 2014). This book presents how Homeopathy as a medical system can contribute to this end of offering a wiser form of healing.

While extolling the virtues of homeopathy and sometimes, appearing to deride allopathy, I wish to inform the reader about what homeopathy is not (Shah, 2011).

1. Homeopathy is not "miracle" medicine – though it can make magical cures for even the most incurable diseases. It is based on certain laws, and there are rules that determine the scope of treatment.

2. It is not a panacea or a cure-for-all, just like other medical practices.

3. It is not just a mind-based medicine, even though emotions and mental states, attitudes, dreams, fears and delusions form an important component in understanding the patient and determining the remedy.

4. It is not some spiritual, soul-based therapy, even though the science of ultra-high dilutions of medicinal substances is still poorly understood by present-day science.

5. It is not some kind of a placebo therapy! As we shall discover later in this book, it works well *in-vitro*, on plants and crops, as well as animals.

CHAPTER 1

Humpty Dumpty's Fall

"When I use a word", Humpty Dumpty said, in rather a scornful tone, "it means just what I choose it to mean—neither more nor less."

– Lewis Carrol: Alice in Wonderland

The Covid-19 pandemic was in many ways a historic watershed event because it exposed the soft underbelly of the modern Western medical system. It exposed the insecurities, fears and weaknesses of a system that has gradually turned into a rigid and ossified institution. A crisis often provides opportunities and moments of change and transformation, but in this crisis, it created new barriers and uncertainties. The enforcement of lockdowns and other restrictions set a new precedent for a militarized response to a civil crisis.

The Humpty Dumpty Effect

As children, all of us learnt the nursery rhyme *Humpty Dumpty* in kindergarten class. Humpty Dumpty was portrayed as a fat, roly-poly, egg shaped character who fell off a wall, had a "great fall", and no one could put him back together again.

However, most of us may not be aware of the real historical Humpty Dumpty. According to several military historians, Humpty Dumpty was the name of a huge cannon installed by the Royalists (King Charles I's Men) on the castle wall in Colchester during the English Civil War to repel the rebel Parliamentarians. The Parliamentarians were the common folk who were fighting for representation rights through a parliament. The canon was short and stubby and apparently, quite unstable. Thus, it was colloquially called "Humpty Dumpty". The rebel forces had damaged a part of the castle wall and when the king's men fired the cannon it rolled over, fell, and broke! Naturally, this was a seen as a great victory of the masses (Parliamentarians), because after the great fall *all the King's Men and all the King's horses couldn't put Humpty Dumpty together again*!

I am going to use the term *Humpty Dumpty Effect* metaphorically, to refer to a situation where a seemingly stable or successful structure or system suddenly collapsed or failed, resulting in significant worldwide chaos. The events that transpired during the Covid-19 pandemic were a metaphorical analogy of the historical Humpty Dumpty event.

This institution was robust, well-funded, well-researched, well-supported by governments and trusted by the populace all the world over. Yet it failed miserably on every front – medical, political, economic and social! The crisis had a dramatic impact on global poverty and inequality. Global poverty increased for the first time in one single generation. The disproportionate income losses among most disadvantaged populations led to a dramatic rise in inequality within and across countries (Sanchez-Pramo, Hill, Mahler, Narayan, & Yonzan, 2021).

So, one may ask, why did the pandemic pan out the way it did? Let us take look at it in greater depth.

The Lancet Fiasco: The canon that came tumbling down

The Lancet, one of the most venerable British peer-reviewed medical journals, formally retracted a paper it had published. The retracted paper was a flawed study on the drug hydroxychloroquine (HCQ). It was originally published on 22 May 2020, and was quickly retracted on June 4, 2020 (Mehra, Desai, & Patel, 2020).

What went wrong?

One of the key findings of the study published was that the use of HCQ actually led to a stunning increase in mortality rates of around 30 percent! This was immediately lapped up by the medical community worldwide. The most familiar face of media and a darling of media houses, Dr. Anthony Fauci, the long-time head of the National Institute of Allergy and Infectious Diseases, confidently announced that *HCQ was "not effective" against coronavirus*, and stopped short of calling for an outright ban (Brennan, 2020). Dr. Fauci was not alone. Eric Topol, a leading American cardiologist also declared that the use of HCQ was associated with a *"significant increase in death."* He was followed by Steven Nissen, a cardiologist at the Cleveland Clinic who said: *"It's a very striking finding and it's convincing to me... Based upon these findings and others, no one should take hydroxychloroquine with or without an antibiotic unless they are in a randomized controlled trial. It should not be used in the general population to prevent or to treat Covid-19 infection."* This was soon followed by bans on the use of HCQ to treat COVID-19 by France, Belgium, and Italy.

Following the dismissal of HCQ, the medical establishment all over the west embraced the use of remdesivir. Remdesivir was an unapproved proprietary drug with possible side effects and no track record of worthwhile benefits. Additionally, remdesivir could only be administered intravenously, rendering it wholly unsuitable for use in underdeveloped countries where the control and treatment of COVID-19 presented a major public health challenge. Therefore, doctors in the United States were prescribing drugs for off-label use and that included extensive use of HCQ to treat Covid-19. The extent of off-label use of drugs for Covid-19 was as high as 50% (Epstein, 2020).

The Humpty Dumpty Effect was in full swing. Doctors were prescribing their own concoctions, with no trials to support other than anecdotal cures. Here is one example. One Dr. Vladimir Zelenko of New York reported that his mix of HCQ, azithromycin and, zinc sulphate was his version of a magical cure. It would have been derided in research circles as an idiosyncratic "snake oil" (Kasprak, 2020). This is one of many examples of reducing medical science to the level of quackery.

The sad part about this is that a respected, peer-reviewed medical journal like *The Lancet* was resorting to political commentary instead of staying with medical science. In its editorial published on 16 May 2020, it strongly advocated that *"Americans must put a President in the White House come January 2021, who will understand that public health should not be guided by partisan politics"* (Lancet, 2020). It is well known that the pharmaceutical industry's funding of election campaigns and lobbying distorts the legislative decisithathich formulate pharmaceutical policies. Hasn't *The Lancet* crossed the red line that every medical journal must strictly observe? We shall deal with this form of corruption in a separate chapter in this book.

CHAPTER 2

Homeopathy in a Pandemic?

"The introduction of homeopathy forced the old-school doctor to stir around and learn something of a rational nature about his business. You may honestly feel grateful that homeopathy survived the attempts of the allopaths to destroy it."

– Mark Twain

The war on Covid was fought by many on numerous fronts. But as the Mayo Clinic admits, *"there is still no cure available for Covid-19"* (MayoClinic, 2023). The mainstay of treatment is treating symptoms with over-the-counter medicines, such as acetaminophen or ibuprofen. The second line of defence was developing a vaccine, and we shall explore that area at length in a later chapter. There was no prophylactic available from the mainstream medicine system. In this state of fear and confusion the spectacular achievements of homeopathy went unnoticed – or rather were purposely and deceitfully suppressed and hidden from the world.

So, what exactly were homeopaths doing across the world in this moment of crisis?

Homeopathy in Epidemics

The Covid-19 pandemic is often compared to the Spanish Flu pandemic of 1918. What is not mentioned in books of medical history is the fact that Homeopathy actually earned its reputation due to its remarkable success in such epidemics. It is interesting to note that homeopaths reported better treatment results as compared to their allopathic counterparts. It turned out to be a deadly disease as its origin and treatment were unknown, yet homeopathy served better than all other treatments known at the time. Likewise, during the nineteenth century, six cholera epidemics plagued Italy and Europe (1834-37, 1848-49, 1854-55, 1865-67, and 1884; 1893). The 19th century saw an explosion of serious epidemic diseases, such as smallpox and scarlet fever, and homeopathy developed a rigorous methodology based on repeated observations in the field, thereby leading to successful results (Negro & Marino, 2021).

During the Spanish Flu epidemic of 1918 homeopaths achieved a strikingly low mortality rate of 2.1 to 5% against 40 to 60% in the case of allopathic treatments. Unfortunately, the censorship of the military institutions, because of the war, did not allow homeopathic doctors of the European countries to publish data about the Spanish flu.

The experience of American homeopaths was much richer and more significant and was widely documented in the *Journal of the American Institute of Homeopathy*. This is confirmed by the article written by Dr. A. Dewey, who collected the case histories of 50 American homeopaths. Their clinical experiences showed an amazing concordance in the percentages of cured cases (90% - 97%) and the remedies used were similar to the Spanish homeopaths but were administered on more cases (Dewey, 1921). In Philadelphia, Dr. Dean W. Pearson collected 26,795 cases treated by various homeopaths, which had much lower mortality of 1.05% compared with 30% of allopaths. In New York, the International Homeopathic Association also reported relevant statistics – 17,000 patients (with many cases of pneumonia) with a mortality of 0.25% (Negro & Marino, 2021).

The success of homeopathy is not restricted to some era in the past. In the year 2007 there was a Chikungunya epidemic across the world.

To deal with this event homeopaths in the State of Kerala, India conducted a cluster-randomised, double-blind, placebo-controlled trial conducted in the 2 districts of Kollam and Alappuzha covering three villages during August-September 2007 (Nair, Gopinadhan, & Kurup, 2014). The homeopathic treatment offered gave a relative risk reduction of 19.7% compared to a relative risk reduction of merely 5.1% by allopathic vaccines.

What was the secret?

Homeopathy uses several approaches for epidemic diseases, and these include individualization, combination remedies, *genus epidemicus*, and isopathy.

Genus epidemicus

Homeopathy has a unique and exceptional approach for finding a remedy suitable for an entire population in an epidemic. Homeopathy does not consider the diagnosis of some specific disease label. When an outbreak of epidemic occurs in a specific area, the first thing homoeopathic doctors do is collect symptoms of the epidemic irrespective of the diagnosis or causative microscopic organisms (e.g., bacteria, viruses, etc.) of the epidemic. As the Founder of Homeopathy, Dr. Samuel Hahnemann said, *"Since every case of disease in a given epidemic has the same origin, the disease puts all those who have fallen ill into the same kind of disease process"*.

A remedy that matches the combined symptoms of a large population afflicted with the same disease or epidemic is called a *genus epidemicus*. If the character of the epidemic disease is discovered according to the symptom complex common to all the patients (i.e. the *genus epidemicus*), this will point to the homeopathically fitting specific remedy for the totality of the cases (Hahnemann, 2013).

The Kerala study mentioned above determined that the *genus epidemicus* for the epidemic of Chikungunya was the remedy Bryonia 30C. The outcomes of its use have been quoted above.

Based on information collected across the country, in January 2020, the Central Council for Homeopathic Research, which works under the Department of Science and Technology, Government of India declared *Arsenicum album* 30C as the *genus epidemicus* for Covid-19. It recommended one dose to be taken on an empty stomach for three days as a prophylactic. A study conducted to audit the efficacy of prophylactic measures against Covid-19 amongst healthcare workers in India found that 24% users were using *Arsenicum album* 30C and fewer that 9.8% tested swab positive (Pillai, Koduri, Gokhale, & Venkatesh, 2021). The vaccine or any other conventional prophylactic drug was still a year and a half away.

But the story of the role of homeopathy does not end here.

CHAPTER 3

Vaccines and Nosodes

"It is not as if our homeopathic brothers are asleep: far from it, they are awake – many of them at any rate – to the importance of the scientific study of disease."

– Sir William Osler, the "Father of Modern Medicine"

The edifice of homeopathy is built on the foundation of the Law of Similars. This Law states that a substance that causes symptoms in a healthy individual when taken in large doses can alleviate those same symptoms in a sick individual when taken in smaller concentrations. This fact was known since the ancient times of Hippocrates (5th century BCE) and the times of Paracelsus (16th century CE). However, Samuel Hahnemann was the first one to actually test this proposition and put it to use it in the clinic, and thereby giving birth to Homeopathy. Hahnemann took 4 drams of cinchona bark (a remedy used in the treatment of malaria) twice a day to test the effects of the drug. What he found was that he developed symptoms like languor, prostration, chills, redness of cheeks, and pulsation in the head – symptoms characteristic of malaria.

The idea of vaccination too, is to an extent, based on the same principle cited above. Edward Jenner who is considered the "father" of the smallpox vaccine was actually following the footsteps of Benjamin Jetsy. Jetsy was a farmer and had discovered this principle by observing that dairymaids on his farm were relatively free from smallpox if they had been infected by cowpox earlier in life. Jetsy therefore rubbed the matter from cowpox pustules into scratches on his skin and later did the same to his wife and son using a darning needle and confirmed this momentous discovery. This happened in 1774, that is 22 years before Jenner did so in 1796 (Pead, 2006).

Jenner had experimentally inoculated just one boy, and on the strength of this single experiment and its questionable interpretation, he based his claim that one vaccination would *"forever secure a person from smallpox"*. That indeed earned him a place in history. The first person experimentally inoculated by Jenner was a young lad named James Phipps. He first injected him with cowpox and six weeks later with smallpox. Later he vaccinated his own son Robert. Tragically, both later died at age 21 and 20 respectively due to tuberculosis. Later on, Jenner's vaccine resulted in numerous other deaths. But these deaths were covered up by recording them as deaths of unvaccinated persons, and the infection cases after vaccination were classified as "pustular eczema" (Humphries & Bystrianyk, 2013).

Measles vaccine

It is well documented that the measles vaccine causes frequent and more severe allergies and autoimmune reactions than other vaccinations. Why is that so? The fact is that the vaccine was developed without isolating the measles virus! This startling discovery was made by a reputed virologist, Dr. Stefan Lanka of Germany. Lanka was the first to discover the maritime virus *Ectocarpus siliculocus* in algae in 1987. During the course of his research he accidentally found that during the development of the measles vaccine there was no evidence that virus had been isolated. The scientific community decided to ignore and sideline him, so he thre a challenge offering a prize of € 100,000 to anyone who could prove him wrong. His offer went unchallenged till one Dr. David

Bardens purportedly produced evidence. In the initial round the Lower Court ruled in favour of Bardens, but the High Court and the Federal Supreme Court ruled in favour of Dr. Lanka and vindicated his stand.

Dr. Stefan Lanka explained his position thus:

"In the trial, the results of research into so-called genetic fingerprints of alleged measles virus have been introduced. Two recognized laboratories, including the world's largest and leading genetic Institute, arrived at exactly the same results independently. The results prove that the authors of the six publications in the measles virus case were wrong, and as a direct result all measles virologists are still wrong today: They have misinterpreted ordinary constituents of cells as part of the suspected measles virus.

"Because of this error, during decades of consensus building process, normal cell constituents were mentally assembled into a model of a measles virus. To this day, an actual structure that corresponds to this model has been found neither in a human, nor in an animal. With the results of the genetic tests, all thesis of existence of measles virus has been scientifically disproved.

"In the trial it was also put on record that the highest German scientific authority in the field of infectious diseases, the RKI, contrary to its legal remit as per § 4 Infection Protection Act (IfSG), has failed to create tests for alleged measles virus and to publish these. This admission may explain the increased rate of vaccination-induced disabilities, namely of vaccination against measles, and why and how specifically this kind of vaccination seems to increasingly trigger autism." (Dmitry, 2017).

What is shameful is the fact that the mainstream media, presumably under pressure and funding from pharmaceutical giants completely blacked out the news of Lanka winning the High Court appeal in 2016 and the 2017 Federal Supreme Court ruling upholding the High Court verdict and also ordered Bardens to bear all procedural costs. Also, no mention is found of the fact that there was no controlled trial of the measles vaccine – ever. A Google search for this matter shows the 2015 lower court ruling favouring Bardens, and the search algorithm drowns the judgements vindicating Lanka.

How does homeopathy overcome such fraud? It can be understood by looking at the basic tenets of homeopathy.

Polio Vaccination: Medicine worse than Disease?

The Vaxxer versus Anti-Vaxxer debate is often an acrimonious discussion that takes place among supporters and opponents of vaccines. A Vaxxer believes that vaccines are safe and should be widely used, while opponents of vaccines believe that they have side effects and risks and that they should not be presented as a sole solution to prevent further outbreaks of infectious diseases. There are also some concerns about the protection provided by vaccines, particularly among vulnerable populations, and about the ethical considerations surrounding vaccination policies.

The best way to have a balanced and intelligent discussion on the topic is to weigh the evidence. Let us take the example of the polio eradication programme in India.

Polio eradication in India has been a remarkable success story. The country launched its polio eradication campaign in 1988, and since then, the number of cases decreased drastically. In 2013 India was declared polio-free by the World Health Organization (WHO), marking a significant milestone in the country's efforts to improve public health. The success of India's polio eradication campaign can be attributed to a combination of factors, including the government's commitment, public awareness programs, and collaboration with various organizations and development partners. However, the statistical success came at a great health and social cost.

According to the World Health Organization, *"There is no cure for polio, it can only be prevented. Polio vaccine, given multiple times, can protect a child for life"* (WHO, 2018). In the year 2000, the WHO recommended that, *"In order to achieve polio eradication in India during 2000, extra national immunization days and house-to-house mopping-up rounds should be organized"*. The polio eradication programme in India was accordingly stepped up vigorously.

If we look at the statistics, it will be seen that the total number of polio cases in India between 1974 to 1993 (ten-year period) numbered 341,000, and the number was declining every year since its peak value of 38,000 cases in 1981 to 4,000 in 1993. The numbers further declined in the next two decades dropping to zero cases in 2011 and 2012, thus leading to the WHO to declare India polio-free in 2013.

What is often overlooked is the fact that this decrease was accompanied with a steady increase in the number of cases of Non-Polio Acute Flaccid Paralysis (NPAFP) in children who were vaccinated. Non-Polio Acute Flaccid Paralysis is characterised by the onset of weakness or paralysis with reduced muscle tone in children. While some cases of flaccid paralysis can be treated, and others may be permanent. Left untreated, the person suffocates due paralysis of the muscles that control breathing. In the State of Uttar Pradesh in India, 35.2% had residual paralysis after 60 days and, alarmingly, 8.5% had died.

In the year 2011 when the last polio case was reported in India, NPAFP rate in India was 13.35 cases per 100,000, whereas the expected rate is only 1 to 2 cases per 100,000. Some states like Uttar Pradesh and Bihar had an APAFP rate as high as 25/100,000 and 35/100,000 respectively. A previous study of data from 2000 to 2010 has detailed the NPAFP rate correlated with the pulse polio rounds conducted there, and the strongest correlation with the NPAFP rate was found when the number of doses from the previous 4 years were used. It has been reported that in 2005 there was a sharp increase in the national NPAFP rate, which coincided with the introduction of a high-potency monovalent vaccine that contained five times the number of Type 1 viruses, compared to that contained in the previously used vaccine (Dhiman, Prakash, Sreenivas, & Puliyel, 2018). In fact, NPAFP rates went down when the oral polio vaccine doses were decreased in 2012.

What is most alarming and yet overlooked by both doctors and administrators is the fact that while the total number of polio cases in the 20-year period from 1974 to 1993 was just 314,000, the NPAFP cases in the 16-year period from 2000 to 2016 was a whopping 642,370 – more than twice the number of polio cases. Sadly, the anticipated fall in the NPAFP rate to 2 per 100,000 has not yet materialized.

This is one example that is well documented, but it points to a major shortcoming, and as Sir Francis Bacon had once said, *the remedy is worse than the disease.*

Therefore, is it not time to explore other possibilities, especially homeopathy?

Law of Similars and Prophylaxis

The development in homeopathy followed a different route. Samuel Hahnemann had discovered that the process of "potentising" a substance actually attenuates its harmful effects and makes it act homeopathically, according to the Law of Similars.

For example, a strong cup of coffee may cause racing thoughts, palpitations, increased urine production, trembling hands, excitability, and restlessness in a healthy person. Drinking coffee before bedtime may also lead to sleep difficulties. However, Hahnemann found that a remedy prepared from coffee could alleviate such symptoms in sick individuals. A hyperactivity child, with agitated thoughts, and sweaty, trembling hands would experience relief with a dose of homeopathic preparation of coffee (*Coffea cruda*). Likewise, *Coffea cruda* may help someone with insomnia caused by racing thoughts and frequent urination. Importantly, not all symptoms may be present for homeopathic treatment to work.

Nosodes

A nosode is one kind of homeopathic medicinal product. It is prepared from diseased human or animal tissues or discharges. The remedy preparation process involves a series of dilutions and succussions. This results in "potentizing" the remedy. Nosodes and vaccines have a lot in common. Some like to call them cousins, or in fact, twins. Both are prepared from biological sources. Vaccines are prepared by weakening the organisms so that they do not retain the toxic or infective properties of the original substance, but still, they have the ability to trigger an immune response that can be protective. Likewise, nosodes retain the immunogenicity to induce an immune response from the human body.

Nosodes are employed in treatment as well as for prophylaxis of disease which exhibit the symptoms similar to symptoms of the disease from which it was sourced. For example, *Hepatitis-C 30C* (Hep C 30), a remedy prepared from HepG2 cells has shown demonstrable anticancer effects against liver cancer cells *in vitro*. The remedy also decreased expression of two cancer biomarkers, Top II and telomerase, consistent with its anticancer effect (Mondal, Das, Shah, & Khudabukhsh, 2016).

Similarly, the remedy *Psorinum 6X* showed evidence of treatment against cancer cells in a controlled study. It inhibited cell proliferation at 24 hours after treatment, and arrested cell cycle at sub-G1 stage. It also induced ROS generation, MMP depolarization, morphological changes and DNA damage, as well as externalization of phosphatidyl serine (Mondal, Samadder, & Khudabukhsh, 2016).

Cuban epidemic: Leptospirosis

Leptospirosis is a zoonotic disease occurring in rainy seasons, which spreads through the urine of domestic and wild animals, and can cause serious infections such as meningitis, hepatitis and pneumonitis. A study was conducted in the year 2007 in three provinces of Cuba where homeo-prophylactic interventions were used.

Homeo-prophylactic formulation from dilutions of four circulating strains of leptospirosis and administered orally to 2.3 million persons at high risk in an epidemic in a region affected by natural disasters. After the homeo-prophylactic intervention, a significant decrease of the disease incidence was observed in the intervention regions compared to the non-intervention regions. The results were re-evaluated, and the findings were consistent with those of the earlier results (Golden & Bracho, 2014).

The Cuban experience created a significant interest internationally among both homoeopaths and the orthodox scientists willing to look at the positive results, even though the mechanism of action was deemed to be 'implausible' according to the orthodox pharmaceutical paradigm.

Dengue outbreak: Delhi 1996

During a dengue outbreak in Delhi in 1996, the Central Council for Research in Homoeopathy distributed *Dengueinum 30* (nosode prepared from the serum of person suffering from dengue fever) to 39,200 people who were not affected and residing in the adversely affected areas for preventing the dengue. A follow-up after 10 days revealed appearance of fever, headache and body ache in five persons only (Nayak & Varanasi, 2020).

Cautions

Nosodes are to be prescribed cautiously as there are some contraindications identified for their prescription. These are as follows:

In the active phase of the disease

During the incubation of the disease

In the acute explosive stage of the disease

During the active phase of a recurrent attack.

In the next chapter we shall see that one homeopath in Mumbai rose to the occasion to pick up the gauntlet during the Covid-19 pandemic.

CHAPTER 4

A Nosode for Covid-19

"If you do not expect the unexpected, you will not find it, for it is not to be reached by search or trail."

– Heraclitus

Dr. Rajesh Shah, MD(Hom) is a successful clinician, author, researcher and a teacher. He has been associated with development of nosodes since the 1996. He is probably the only homeopathic researcher who has worked in close association with cytogeneticists and molecular biologists. His research in collaboration with leading molecular biologists like Dr. AR Khuda-Bukhsh, as well as other scientists at the Tata Memorial Advanced Centre for Treatment, Research and Education in Cancer (ACTRECT) has shown not only the efficacy but also the mechanism of action of the nosodes. He has published over 35 peer reviewed papers and led research to discover fifteen new drugs.

The HIV virus was discovered by Luc Antoine Montagnier and his team sometime around 1981, which made Dr. Shah immediately think of making the *HIV Nosode*. It took him about 30 years to develop *HIV Nosode* in 2008-2009. The nosode *HIV 30C* prevented cancer cell proliferation and migration, induced pre-mature senescence, enhanced pro-apoptotic signal proteins like p53, bax, cytochrome c, caspase-3 and inhibited anti-apoptotic signal proteins Bcl2, TERT and Top II, changed mitochondrial membrane potential and caused externalization of phosphatidyl serine (Khuda-Bukhsh, Mondal, & Shah, 2017).

Later, Dr. Shah went on to develop about twelve new nosodes and conduct scientific research using modern techniques. Some of these nosodes are prepared from organisms such as *HIV, Hepatitis C, Mycobacterium Tuberculosis, E Coli, Plasmodium falciparum, HPV, Salmonella,* and *Cancer* tissues, etc. Dr. Shah likes to describe nosodes as "homeopathically prepared oral vaccines at room temperature" (RajGuru, In Conversation with Dr. Rajesh Shah – The Developer of a COVID-19 Nosode, 2021).

Covid-19 Nosode development

The nosode was developed from 3 variants of COVID-19 nosodes at the BSL2 facility at Haffkine Institute, Mumbai and Gujarat University, by end of May and July 2020. One variant was from a clinical sample containing a live virus, another from certain inactivated strains, and the third from spike glycoproteins (Shah, 2020). All safety precautions applicable to modern vaccine development were strictly followed, even though preparation of a nosode involves serial dilution beyond the Avogadro's number and in fact, no RNA material exists beyond 5C potency. In line with conventional guidelines, OECD/ NDCT guidelines for animal toxicity testing were followed. For the first time these guidelines were observed in nosode studies to facilitate rapid acceptance to conventional standards. Similarly, strict, conventional standards were applied for in-vitro studies.

Phase 1 studies were conducted on 10 healthy volunteers under ICMR guidelines. None of the volunteers developed any serious adverse effects. Drug proving symptoms were documented. What is particularly noteworthy is that all the 10 volunteers showed an elevation of certain cytokines thereby suggesting immune response in the form of T-cell activation. Also, there was an increase in CD4 count in 70% of the volunteers. Thus, perhaps for the first time it was demonstrated that a homeopathic potency of 30C can elicit an immune response. This finding itself presents another opportunity to explore how such an ultra-dilute dose could retain the ability to induce an immune response.

Observational Clinical Trial

After that, an observational clinical trial was conducted. The Municipality of Mumbai was running many quarantine facilities, so Dr. Shah's team collaborated with them, and trials were conducted in one such facility housing more than 2,200 high-risk individuals who had been exposed. The placebo-controlled multi-arm clinical trial was completed on 2,233 people. The nosode was compared with other indicated homeopathic remedies like *Arsenicum album*, *Bryonia*, and *Camphora*, with about 325 persons in each of the six arms. In this human study, Covid-19 nosode showed 62% efficacy against placebo.

Compare this with the fact that the combined efficacy of full vaccination was at 44.5% for preventing asymptomatic infections as was reported by *The Lancet Microbe* in a meta-analysis of 27 RCTs. In fact, vaccine efficacy against symptomatic infection waned over time after full vaccination, with an average decrease of 13.6% per month and had to be enhanced by a booster. (Yang, Jiang, Li, & Zhao, 2023).

At the time of writing the Covid-19 nosode has successfully completed phase 2 and phase 3 trials with unprecedented findings and is posed to be posed to be a gamechanger. That is because unlike vaccines, nosodes can be used for a host of other diseases and pathologies.

For example, *Syphilinum*, a remedy prepared from syphilitic virus, has been found to be effective in osteoporosis (Saha, 2010). But it is also well known for its beneficial action on body tissues wherever the destructive process is present. Apart from its universal healing action to stop the destruction of body tissues, *Syphilinum* is of great help in treating bone necrosis. The most dominant feature for selecting *Syphilinum* in any given case of Avascular Necrosis is the "worsening of bone pains at night". The person experiences pain throughout the night and is unable to sleep on account of the severe pain. The pains may compel the patient to walk, which seems to bring relief. Such persons remain comparatively well the whole day (Allen H. , 2007).

It would be incorrect to think that since *Syphilinum* is prepared from the syphilis virus it would act against that disease. When a poison is potentized the essential character of the molecules is undoubtedly lost, and hence it is not the same substance any longer. Therefore, there can be no certainty that the potentized preparation is the same poison.

Sadly, new homeopathic drug regulation is not well-defined in most parts of the world, and as a result, these new drugs cannot be made available for mass use. Dr. Shah has been working on this issue for over a decade and hopes to see the approval process in place in the near future. *Syphilinum* works in a wide range of conditions, ranging from acute ophthalmia, hereditary tendency to alcoholism, profuse leucorrhoea, obstinate constipation, and so many more diverse conditions.

CHAPTER 5

A Rainbow of Lies

"In questions of science, the authority of a thousand is not worth the humble reasoning of a single individual."

– Galileo Galilei

Looking out for a rainbow when the sun breaks out of the clouds is what all of us love to do. Indeed, some do find the rainbow in the horizon, while others find a metaphorical equivalent by peering down a microscope to search life, or by looking into the dark sky searching nebulae and star bursts creating matter. However, those who do not have an eye for wonder are left to look at mere numbers, and unfortunately miss the rainbow. But very often readers, be they laypersons or even clinicians, are confused by numbers and statistics.

The image of scientists as objective seekers of truth is periodically jeopardized by the discovery of a major scientific fraud. Recent scandals have shown how easy it can be for a scientist to publish fabricated data in the most prestigious journals, and how this can cause a waste of financial and human resources and might pose a risk to human health.

So, how frequent are scientific frauds? The question is very crucial.

The frequency with which scientists fabricate and falsify data or commit other forms of scientific misconduct is a matter of controversy. Many surveys have asked scientists directly whether they have committed or know of a colleague who committed research misconduct, but their results appeared difficult to compare and synthesize.

The US Federal Drug Administration has admitted that from 1977 to 1990, between 10% to 20% of all studies were flawed. In 33.7% of cases, data or results had been fabricated, falsified or modified. Other questionable research practices were found in 72% of the papers! Sadly, misconduct was reported more frequently by medical and pharmacological researchers than others (Fanelli, 2009).

Scientific results can be distorted in several ways. Data can be "cooked", the object of which is to give to ordinary observations the appearance and character of those of the highest degree of accuracy. Or it can be "mined" to find a statistically significant relationship that is then presented as the original target of the study; or, it can be selectively published only when it supports one's expectations. It can also conceal conflicts of interest. These misbehaviours are part of the rainbow of lies that covers scientific fraud, bias, and sometimes, simple carelessness. They are be covered under an innocent sounding phrase – "questionable research practices" or QRP for short. Between 6.2% and 72% of respondents of a survey conducted by Fanelli had knowledge of various QRPs.

Indeed, there are a few students and scientists who accept negative results of their experiments and make major discoveries. But by and large, everyone thinks that negative results are meaningless and does not advance their career.

Replication crisis in medicine

Replicability or reproducibility in science refers to the ability to reproduce research findings consistently in different experiments or studies. This is a critical component of scientific integrity and helps to establish the validity and reliability of research results. Replicability issues can arise due to a variety of factors, such as experimental error, biased sampling, or variations in research techniques. To address these issues, researchers are increasingly employing open science practices, such as sharing their data and methods, to promote transparency and reproducibility in scientific research.

Many studies claim a significant result, but their findings cannot be reproduced. This problem has attracted increased attention in recent years, with several studies providing evidence that research is often not reproducible. A 2016 survey by the reputed journal *Nature*, for example, revealed that in the field of biology alone, over 70% of researchers were unable to reproduce the findings of other scientists and approximately 60% of researchers could not reproduce their own findings (Baker, 2016).

The attitude of researchers is quite varied towards these findings. More than half (52%) of those surveyed agree that there is a significant 'crisis' of reproducibility.

Dr. John Ioannidis is a Stanford professor and a widely cited scientist, with more than 360,000 citations and has published over 1000 research papers. He says that science has grown *"from the occupation of a few dilettanti into a vibrant global industry"* with more than 15 million people authoring more than 25 million scientific papers between 1996–2011 alone (Ioannidis, 2014). However, true and readily applicable major discoveries are far fewer. Currently, an estimated 85% of research resources are wasted (Macleod, et al., 2014).

What is more shocking is the fact that published papers that fail to replicate are cited more than those that replicate - even after the failure is published (Serra-Garcia & Gneezy, 2021). As you may be aware, the number of citations is a basic measure that is used to assess the scholarly impact of a published work. Why are non-replicable papers accepted for publication in the first place? A possible answer is that the review team faces a trade-off. When the results are more "interesting," they apply lower standards regarding their reproducibility – it is a true "marriage of convenience".

I have just cited two publications, but these are not exceptional findings. Top medical journals, which include the *BMJ*, *Lancet*, and the *New England Journal of Medicine (NEJM)*, all have reported this time and again.

For example, Maria Angell, the first woman Editor-in-Chief of *NEJM* mentions in her book, *Science on Trial*, that in many medical specialties where drugs are frequently used, it is difficult to find an expert who does not have financial ties to at least one drug company. This could lead to potential conflicts of interest and raise questions about the objectivity of medical advice and treatment recommendations. Angell has described the pharmaceutical industry "awash with money" and as being the most profitable industry since the 1980s.

Richard Horton, the Editor-in-Chief of *The Lancet* is quite forthright in stating that *"Journals have devolved into information laundering operations for the pharmaceutical industry"* (Horton, 2014).

Richard Smith, former Editor-in-Chief of *The BMJ* who served for 25 years, argues that medical journals, particularly those that receive funding from pharmaceutical companies, are often used as a tool for marketing drugs. He suggests that these journals selectively publish studies that show a positive outcome for the drug, while suppressing or negatively reporting studies that show otherwise. This, in turn, can create a false sense of security for doctors and patients who rely on these journals as a source of medical information. He states, *"I must confess that it took me almost a quarter of a century editing for the BMJ to wake up to what was happening. Medical journals are an extension of the marketing arm of pharmaceutical companies"* (Smith, 2005).

Science by consensus?

Consensus has no value in a scientific argument; because consensus, by definition is about congruity of opinion, and not empirical evidence.

Science by consensus is a disturbing trend where scientific ideas or conclusions are reached based on a group agreement rather than rigorous scientific evidence. Sadly, this trend has become increasingly common, as it undermines the core principles of scientific inquiry and jeopardizes the credibility and objectivity of scientific research. Consensus is not a substitute for scientific evidence, and scientists must adhere to rigorous research methods and peer review to ensure the integrity of their findings.

Among the highly contested issues are genetically modified (GM) crops, vaccines, endocrine-disrupting chemicals, pesticides, cell phone electromagnetic emissions, salt intake, obesity, smokeless tobacco, electronic cigarettes, particulate air pollution, hydraulic fracturing ("fracking") to extract natural gas, and climate change.

Take climate change, for example. We are told that there is an overwhelming "consensus" among scientists that climate change is man-made and is likely to have catastrophic effects over the coming century. Yet, the American Medical Association *"supports the findings of the Intergovernmental Panel on Climate Change's fourth assessment report and concurs with the **scientific consensus** that the Earth is undergoing adverse global climate change and that anthropogenic contributions are significant"* (AMA, 2022). A question of such a staggering complexity has been reduced to a binary choice between two extremes, either climate change is a "hoax" or is an unquestionable certainty. Effectively, the claim of a 97% consensus is political and is directed at the lay public, who may know little about the science but who, understandably, react to frightening scenarios involving impending catastrophe. There are no controlled studies that allow us to isolate the effects of a human intervention contributing to the effect (Kabat, 2017).

Consensus – Spicy food causes ulcers!

There was a scientific consensus for centuries on abdominal ulcers. That was, *"Ulcers are caused primarily by stress and spicy food"*. But it took the research and study of two researchers, Barry Marshall and Robin Warre, who found in 1982 that the real cause was a bacteria called *Helicobacter pylori*. They won the Nobel Prize for this discovery in 2005. The Gram negative curved bacillus *H. pylori* then became the prize bug of all times! They had found that more than 90% of duodenal ulcers and up to 80% of gastric ulcers are caused by this bacillus. Yet, the clinical community met their findings with scepticism and a lot of criticism and that's why it took quite a remarkable length of time for their discovery to become widely accepted. That is the influence of a popular consensus over scientific discovery.

But there is a twist in the tale! A bacterium that was existing in human stomachs for hundreds of thousands of years must have had a purpose beyond making people sick? Was there a possible symbiotic relationship? That has been debated since the discovery of this pathogen. However, the debate has been intensified in the past few years as some studies have posed the possibility that the infection may be beneficial in some humans. Strong evidence suggests that absence of *H. pylori* from the stomach may lead to cancers of other gut regions, and that *H. pylori* infection in fact protects against gastro-oesophageal reflux (Ahmed, 2005).

Medical Science and Physics Envy

Physics has dominated the field of science in the last 200 years and indeed the discoveries of physics are spectacular. But unwittingly it has led to a rush in other sciences, such as medicine, psychology, anthropology, sociology, economics and a host of other fields of enquiry to copy and ape physics. This is now officially known as Physics Envy. Physics has long been regarded as the model of what a science should be. Perhaps it started with Descartes who famously said, *"God created the world as a perfect clockwork mechanism, … you understand the parts and you understand the whole."*

It has been the hope, and the expectation, that if sufficient time, resources and talent need to be put into the sciences concerned with other phenomena—in particular the life sciences and the behavioural and social sciences. It is now presumed that that all good science should be "physics-like", that is, distinguished by quantitative specification of every phenomena, mathematical sharpness and deductive power of the theory that is used to explain these phenomena. Indeed, Galileo had famously said that the universe is written in the language of mathematics.

Life sciences, and medicine in particular, was not afflicted with this malady of Physics Envy a century ago, and it may be attributed to the Flexner Report that was published sometime in 1910. It transformed the nature and process of medical education in America, and consequently in the rest of the world where medical education was following the western model. The report had its origins in the enchantment of Mr. Abraham Flexner with German medical education. Flexner was a former schoolteacher and expert on educational practices but had no background in medicine! Flexner himself was surprised about his appointment to this position, suspecting that he was being confused with his brother, Simon, who was a doctor.

At the time of his appointment, the former high school teacher had never been inside a medical school (Duffy, 2011). What was most damaging in the Flexner Report was his omission of any consideration of a physician's healing role and how education should foster that art. This has resulted in a hyper-rationalized medicine and in fact went against the wisdom of Sir Willian Osler, the father of modern medicine, which gave primacy to the beneficence of the patient. A delicate balance of patient care and research could have been pursued with mutual benefits for both sides, but that was overlooked by the schoolmaster to the detriment of the practice of medicine and the attitude of the medical establishment in the century that followed.

The requirement to conform to standards of physics overlooks the complexity in life sciences. Only measurables are considered relevant.

For example, subjective parameters like feelings and emotions are not considered. As a matter of fact, Richard Feynmann, one of the great scientists of the last century who had an inimitable style of teaching had famously said, "Imagine how much harder physics would be if electrons had feelings". What he was trying to say is that the methods of physics and mathematics do not apply all sciences. In this context, Prof. Andrew Lo of the MIT Sloan School of Management laments that, *"All sciences want to reduce 99% of their observations to just three laws, but the sad reality is that most often in complex sciences there may be 99 laws to explain just 3% of the stuff!"* (Lo & Mueller, 2010). Even a wise man like Earnest Rutherford, who won the Nobel Prize for physics in 1909 held the view that, *"All science is either physics or stamp collection"* (Wolf, Katsnelson, & Koonin, 2018).

In view of the above there are some winds of change that are visible. It is being recognised that this uncertainty in medicine need not be viewed as a constraint, rather it should be embraced because of the opportunity it provides doctors and patients to engage on more profound levels and reflect on alternative possibilities. Homeopathy is often criticised or even ridiculed because the miraculous results cannot be understood with the present models of reductionist, physics-envy driven thought.

Some authors like Caroline Wellbery extol the value of uncertainty. Wellbery, in her essay Art of Medicine in *The Lancet* cautions that "in a world of increasing medical knowledge, capabilities, and expectations, the extent of uncertainty is rarely discussed, despite findings that one in three necropsies disagreed with the stated cause of death." Practitioners should use ambiguity in medical practice as an impetus to gain greater certainty about other facets of a patient (Lancet, 2010). This is something homeopathy has incorporated from the time of its inception. The entire science and practice of homeopathy is patient centric and individualised.

'Extremely Productive' (EP) Authors

Authorship is the coin of scholarship — and some researchers are literally "minting" a lot. Ioannidis and his co-researchers randomly searched Scopus for authors who had published more than 72 papers (the equivalent of one paper every 5 days!) in any one calendar year between 2000 and 2016, a figure that many would consider implausibly prolific (Ioannidis, Klavans, & Boyack, 2018). They counted more than 9,000 individuals, who had submitted 'full papers' — not articles, conference papers, substantive comments and reviews, nor editorials, letters to the editor and the like. Alarmingly, up to four times more researchers pump out more than 60 papers a year than less than a decade ago. Naturally, the increase in these 'extremely productive' authors raises concerns that some researchers are resorting to dubious methods to publish extra papers. What is more shocking is that overall, most EP authors outside physics were in clinical medicine. Saudi Arabia had the highest number of EP authors followed by Italy.

"Something is wrong in medicine"

Let us take the example of a drug called Reboxetine. It serves as an example of one of the many problems with how drugs are developed. Reboxetine (known commercially as Edronax) is an antidepressant. Many psychiatrists prescribe it because the published scientific evidence showed that it is quite effective. The problem is that doctors are often misled. In this case, a total of seven trials pitting Reboxetine against placebo had been run. All except for one had shown no difference between the two. But the only trial whose results were actually published was the one showing Reboxetine was better than placebo (Goldacre, 2013).

In other words, out of six negative trials and one positive trial, the negative trials were buried and didn't see the light of day until a research team unearthed them. This is one of the major problems with the pharmaceutical industry: there are tremendous incentives to only publish the results of clinical trials that favour them and to never share the results of negative trials. This skewing of the medical literature necessarily impacts the decisions doctors make. How can a physician judge the true worth of a drug when the portrait that emerges from the literature has been doctored?

Opioid crisis and lives in danger

A new public health crisis that has emerged as a byproduct of medical care itself is the opioid crisis. The opioid crisis is the latest self-inflicted wound of the healthcare system. In the US alone, there were 240 million opioid prescriptions dispensed in 2015, nearly one for every adult in the general population (Makary, 2017). Too many people are leaving hospital with bottles of opioid tablets they don't need. As of 2018, 128 Americans die each day of an opioid overdose, and total economic costs associated with opioid misuse are estimated to be more than $500 billion annually. The crisis has evolved in three phases, starting in the 1990s and continuing through 2010 with a massive increase in use of prescribed opioids associated with lax prescribing regulations and aggressive marketing efforts by the pharmaceutical industry. Since 2013, the third phase of the crisis has included a movement towards synthetic opioids, especially fentanyl (Maclean, Mallat, Ruhm, & Simon, 2020).

Unfortunately, homeopathy is often overlooked as a modality for pain management. However, it deserves to be a first-line treatment due to its safety, effectiveness, and cost-effectiveness. The database of the social security system in France, where citizens can choose a homeopathic or conventional family doctor, shows that homeopathy provides comparable results in pain management while significantly reducing the use of conventional painkillers. Sadly, the resistance to the use of homeopathy is based on the mistaken notion that it contains nothing but water!

A Picture is Worth a Thousand Lies!

Dr. Elisabeth Bik, a Dutch-born US-based microbiologist is a "science integrity consultant". She worked 15 years in the School of Medicine at Stanford, on the microbiomes of humans and marine mammals. In May 2014, she founded *Microbiome Digest*, a daily compilation of scientific papers in the rapidly growing microbiome field. She worked as a Science Editor at *uBiome* and was later the Scientific and Editorial Director.

Bik has a remarkable natural ability to identify both image duplication and image manipulation through visual screening and has been described as a "champion spotter" of duplicated or altered images. One of her most celebrated cases is that of Khalid Shah, a top neuroscientist at Harvard Medical School who allegedly falsified data and plagiarized images across 21 papers (Paulus & Ravi, 2024). According to Bik, she started her investigation following a tip from someone who was familiar with Shah's laboratory. She investigated potential research misconduct and claimed to find image reuse or duplication problems across 29 papers, which he published in 21 different journals between 2001 and 2024. Shah is listed as the first, second, or corresponding author on 25 of the 29 papers (Gerhard, 2024).

Bik contributed to data falsification allegations against four top scientists at the Dana-Farber Cancer Institute – leading to the retraction of six, and correction of 31 papers – and independently reviewed research misconduct allegations against former Stanford President Marc T. Tessier-Lavigne, which played a part in his resignation later.

Short "lifespan" of Drugs

Drugs are developed by the pharmaceutical companies and the only way to offset the cost of research is to market such patented drugs at a price that recovers the amount invested in the shortest period of time. New drugs are often hailed as the poster child for the proposition that patents encourage accelerated rates of innovation. This sentiment derives, in large part, from the belief that pharmaceutical research and development (R&D) entails significant costs and resources. What is not revealed is the fact that it is the cost of marketing, advertisement and incentives offered to doctors for prescribing are the largest contributors that inflate the cost far more than R&D costs (Basheer, 2012). Also, it is the market demand rather than health needs that drives drug research. Contrary to popular belief, the overall investment in drug research and development is too low, compared with profits (Barton & Emanuel, 2005).

Despite the high investments and even greater profits raked in by the powerful pharmaceutical companies, drugs that are made to save lives cause death. Every year medicines are withdrawn from the market due to adverse drug reactions, often resulting in death. Hepatic, cardiac, seizures, heart valve damage, veno-occlusive disease, bone marrow suppression, aplastic anaemia, and nervous system toxicity are the principal reasons for withdrawals (Igho, Carl, & Aronson, 2016).

Contrast this with the fact that in its two and a half centuries of existence, not a single homeopathic remedy has ever been banned due to adverse drug reaction and the drug development cost by *provings* or HPT are minuscule.

CHAPTER 6

Future in the Past

"Medicine is a science of uncertainty and an art of probability."

– Sir William Osler, MD
Father of Modern Western Medicine

"Future in the past" is a common phrase used in science fiction novels and films. It refers to the concept of traveling back in time to change the course of the future. Sometimes called "time travel," this idea is based on the theory that the past and future are interconnected, and our actions in the present can affect both. In the world of science fiction, the possibilities of what could happen if we were able to visit the future and alter it are endless. However, in our reality, time travel has not yet been invented, but in medical science we have already achieved that to some extent!

Medicine in the Future refers to advances in medical technology and treatment methods that are expected to be available in the future. These developments are aimed at improving health outcomes, reducing the burden of disease, and increasing overall wellness. Some of the potential areas of focus for future medicine include, (a) precision medicine, (b) personalized treatment, (c) targets genetic disposition, and (d) preventive medicine.

Is there a system of medicine that already has all the four ingredients mentioned?

Presently, the only system of medicine that is precise, personalised, considers genetic disposition, and acts as a preventative is Homeopathy, and it has been around since the nineteenth century – a perfect example of "future in the past". It addresses both acute and chronic diseases, speeds recovery in surgical cases and works wonders in epidemics. However, unscientific, and biased points of view have stunted its growth and integration into current pharmaceutical industry driven western medical system. For nearly two centuries Homeopathy-bashing has served both as a hobby and a life-support to many who have lived on the pickings of the allopathic-pharmaceutical complex. This works both at the gross as well as subtle level.

Criticism

In the year 2015 Australian National Health and Medical Research Council (NHMRC) issued a statement that there is no "good quality evidence" to support the claim that homeopathy is effective in treating health conditions. The conclusions of this report were allegedly based on a "rigorous assessment" of 1,800 papers. However, it was admitted that out of these only 225 studies met the criteria to be included in NHMRC's examination of the effectiveness of homeopathy.

Let us take a look at the members of the Homeopathic Working Committee of NHMRC which prepared the report. Of the seven members, only one member, Prof. Peter Brooks MBBS, MD, had a background in Complementary and Alternative Medicine. For reasons unexplained, Dr. Brooks was *required to step down* from the Chairmanship of HWC. Was it because he had in the past been associated with setting up the Australian Centre for Complementary Medicine Education and Research at the University of Queensland, in association with Southern Cross University? All discussions were purported to be *robust and open*, yet ironically decision-making was majority-based, with no reference to dissent – thus ensuring that any sane voice would be drowned in the din of a motivated majority (NHMRC, 2015).

Turning a Blind Eye

The report also admits that it did not consider any evidence from (a) laboratory studies, (b) studies in animals, (c) studies in humans without a specific health condition; nor did it focus on the safety of homeopathic medicines. It did not take into consideration any personal testimonials as the HWC opined that they are not reliable as people may experience health benefits because they "believe that a treatment is effective". So, they relied on "evidence-based methods", in particular the Randomized Controlled Trials (RCTs) as they are claimed to be the "gold standard" for testing medical efficacy. For that reason, NHMRC did not consider observational studies, individual experiences and testimonials, case series and reports, or research that was not done using standard methods (NHMRC, 2015). This is quite strange because traditionally, surgeons have relied principally on three types of research, namely, animal experiments, case reports and case series only (Jones, 2013).

RCTs - Gold Standard or the Golden Calf?

The Golden Calf is a famous biblical story in the Book of Exodus, Chapter 32 in which the Israelites turned away from God and created a statue of a golden calf to worship and replace Moses, who had led them out of Egypt. After an idol maker named Aaron crafted the statue and the Israelites began to worship it, God became angry and threatened to destroy them. The double-blind randomized controlled trial (RCT) is widely accepted by medicine as objective scientific methodology. When ideally performed, it produces knowledge untainted by bias stands. But today RCTs stand at a crossroad where serious doubts about potential biases such as "preference" or "investigator self-selection" are suggesting unethical and corrupt practices and mimic the worship of the Golden Calf.

In recent times, even such respected and conservative (and not-so-well-disposed-to-Homeopathy) journals such as *The Lancet* have been questioning the faith placed in RCTs and pointing to its serious limitations. One scholar admits that *"RCTs most often lack evidence that the treatment under investigation will prove of any use to a real patient seen by a doctor in the clinic* (Rothwell, 2005). *The ritualistic worship of RCTs comes in for critical comment in a McGill University paper which concludes that, "the legitimacy of Evidence Based Medicine relies neither on experts nor numbers, but on distinct procedures for handling (non) Evidence, reflecting its 'regulatory objectivity'"* (Knappen, 2013). In a textbook on RCTs, Jadad and Enkin admonish us *"to stop worshiping the randomized controlled trial as if it were a talisman that would guarantee objectivity"*. As early as 1998, Rene Favaloro, the father of coronary artery bypass surgery (CABG) had warned against the *"almost religious sanctification"* of the ideology of RCTs (Jones, 2013). That is so because RCTs do a good job to solve simple or complicated problems but have very limited use in complex problems like human health and well-being. To cite an example, raising a child and treating dementia would hardly lend itself to RCTs (Jadad & Enkin, 2007). In its wisdom NHMRC chose to turn a blind eye to these realities.

How does homeopathy avoid such occurrences?

Homoeopathic Pathogenetic Trials (HPTs)

Homeopathic pathogenetic trial (HPT), also known as a *Drug proving* is a process unique to Homeopathy. It is a scientific process in which drug substances are put into trial on healthy human volunteers and their pathogenetic effects are observed, noted and compiled. Unlike conventional medicine where animal experimentation forms the basis of evaluation of drug pathogenesis, homoeopathic medicines are proved on healthy human volunteers, including controls, from both sexes and age group. Provings have been the mainstay in homeopathic practice since its inception. Dr. Samuel Hahnemann, the Founder of Homeopathy, carried out the first HPT with *Cinchona officinalis*, a common remedy in his times for malaria, and recorded the pathogenesis of the drug. The symptoms that developed in him in a state of health bore great similarity to malarial fever. This led Hahnemann to theorise that the specific curative power of a drug could lie in its ability to produce symptoms similar to the disease it could cure (Hahnemann, 2013). Since the times of Hahnemann, HPTs have been regarded as the best way of obtaining an unadulterated picture of a drug. Once a drug proving has elicited the symptoms generated, the next step is introducing the remedy into clinical practice and confirming its efficacy. The method is completely replicable.

Sadly, within the current regulations, homeopathic drug proving trials are classified as phase 1 trials, although their aim is not to explore the safety and pharmacological dynamics of the drug, but rather to find clinical indications according to the theory of homeopathy. During an HPT, to avoid bias, it is necessary that neither the subjects nor the investigators know the identity of the drug. This requires a modification to the informed consent process and blinded study materials. Because it is impossible to distinguish between adverse events and proving symptoms, both must be documented together, because the toxic effects of the drug serve as the key source of information for the homeopathic materia medica and guide to clinical use.

HPTs have evolved tremendously since the times of Hahnemann. Today, the same rigorous standards of double-blinded RCTs are applied to all drug provings. However, there is a rich texture in terms of the data that is collected. What is collected is actually a high-resolution portrait of drug-triggered pathogenesis as it covers the locality of the symptoms, the associated sensations, modalities (factors which aggravate or ameliorate), concomitants (symptoms that typically accompany other symptoms), times when symptoms appear or disappear, moods and emotional states of mind experienced and clinical findings. The final part is conducted when the drug identity has been revealed at the end of the trial. The results will then be related to the traditional and scientific knowledge available on the drug being investigated and discussed in the research team before being introduced in the materia medica and used in the clinic.

There is a new trend that underlines the necessity of including the importance of disease-producing power or pathogenesis of the substance being proved while testing suitability as a remedy. This is especially important if remedies have to be developed for specific disease.

Thus, it will be seen that HPTs have an inherent built-in safety mechanism to prevent fraud, and are 100% replicable. Also, homeopathic medicines in their pure form are not patentable, which leads to another benefit: they are extremely inexpensive.

Homeopathy foresaw the role of the human microbiome

The human organism and the human microbiome work as a complex super-organism throughout the human lifecycle. Microbiome science provides direct evidence and substantiation of the fundamental principles of homeopathy, including holism, psychosomatics, direction of cure, the Law of Similars, individuality and susceptibility, minimum dose, and homeostasis. Many conventional allopathic medical treatments irreversibly damage the ecology of the microbiome and trigger chronic immune dysfunction and inflammation. As a consequence, the future sustainability of the entire field of medicine depends on the ability to recognize these inconvenient biological truths and to embrace a safer approach based on this evidence. Fortunately, one of the oldest forms of clinically verifiable, evidence-based, and ecologically sustainable medicine, which does not harm the microbiome, already exists in the form of homeopathy (Whitmont, 2020).

Research has determined that there are more than ten thousand different microbial species and more than 100 trillion different individual organisms colonizing the average normal healthy human body. In fact, individual "non-human" micro-organisms in the human microbiome outnumbers human cells and weighs almost 1.5 kilogrammes (Gorman, 2003). The human microbiome is a unified whole, and function as an independent, inter-connected, invisible, essential "organ" throughout the human body. It plays a critical role in metabolism, development, and homeostasis, and directly modulates the host inflammatory immune response.

Bowel nosodes: Homeopathic foresight into gut microbiota

Gut bacteria are an important component of the microbiota ecosystem in the human gut, which is colonized by 100 trillion microbes - more than the total number of human cells! Gut bacteria play an important role in human health, such as supplying essential nutrients, synthesizing vitamin K, aiding in the digestion of cellulose, and promoting angiogenesis and enteric nerve function. However, they can also be potentially harmful due to the change of their composition when the gut ecosystem undergoes abnormal changes in the light of the use of antibiotics, illness, stress, aging, bad dietary habits, and lifestyle. Dysbiosis of the gut bacteria communities can cause many chronic diseases, such as inflammatory bowel disease, obesity, cancer, and autism (Zhang, et al., 2015).

One of the failings of Western medicine over the last century has been a tendency to over-rationalise illness around mechanistic models of causation. The state of illness is actually a set of complex dynamic reactions and counter-reactions. These are brought about by intimate relationships that exist between individual organisms, within groups of organisms and within/ between species. Overlooking this fact makes modern medicine rather unidimensional. Today, it is accepted that gut microbiota can be best understood as a hidden metabolic organ because it has an immense impact on human wellbeing, including host metabolism, physiology, nutrition and immune function. Our gut microbiome co-evolves with us, and any disharmonious changes can lead to conditions such as obesity, malnutrition, diabetes, and chronic inflammatory diseases such as ulcerative colitis, Crohn's disease etc. (Guinane & Cotter, 2013).

For example, it is now an accepted scientific fact that specific infective agent (bacteria, fungi, viruses), in many cases of disease, can be isolated and identified. But is it a true conclusion that the specific infective agent is always the cause of the disease? Dr. John Paterson, a British researcher, continuing the work of Dr. Edward Bach, a research bacteriologist made some startling discoveries. He found that *B. coli*, a type of bacteria found in the intestines of humans and animals, is a normal part of the gut's microbiome, but it can also cause food poisoning and other illnesses.

How can a normally resident bacteria be both poisonous and a harmless passenger in the gut? He examined more than 20,000 stool specimens and his research spanned over 20 years. He found that bowel flora to be a harmless saprophyte (an organism that obtains food by consuming dead or decaying organic matter from plants and animals). Also, it was non-pathogenic in the healthy bowel. Its function is to break up into simpler substances the complex molecules of the organic combinations, which form the bodies of plants and animals, or of the complex substances which result from the digestive processes in the intestinal canal and are excreted. However, in sickness and disease, the very same bacteria turn pathogenic. Paterson and Bach asked the vital question, "Is the *specific germ* the actual cause of disease, or is it the result of the action of the Vital Force (which characterises all living cells), in their resistance to disease?" Indeed, each germ is associated with its own peculiar symptom picture of disease and that certain conclusions may be made from these clinical and laboratory observations and translated into the practice of medicine (Paterson, 2017).

This reminds one of the prophetic words of Dr. James Tyler Kent (1849-1916), an eclectic doctor who later turned homeopath. He famously said that *"In the course of time we will be able to show perfectly that the microscopical little fellows are not the disease cause, but that they come after, that they are scavengers accompanying the disease, and that they are perfectly harmless in every respect. They are the outcome of the disease, are present wherever the disease is, and by the microscope it has been discovered that every pathological result has its corresponding bacteria."* (Kent, 2008).

A major discovery that Dr. Edward Bach and Dr. John Paterson made was that the potentised homeopathic remedies affected the appearance or disappearance of these non-lactose fermenting bacilli. In the laboratory they observed an unexpected phenomenon, that from a patient who had previously yielded only *B. Coli* there suddenly appeared a large percentage of non-lactose fermenting bacilli of a type which one associated with the pathogenic group of typhoid and paratyphoid.

If one were to accept the view that is generally held, that the *B. Coli* of the intestinal tract is a harmless saprophyte and is non-pathogenic it must be concluded that, so far as the intestinal tract was concerned there was no evidence of disease in these patients during the first series of examinations. Now the patient's stool yielded a large percentage of *presumably* pathogenic organisms, and according to the accepted Pasteur and Koch theory, the patient was suffering from disease. Clinical investigations, however, revealed that the patient did not feel ill, but had experienced a sense of wellbeing which he had attributed to the last medicine he had received. The pathogenic germ in this case was the result of the action set up by the Vital Force in the patient by the potentized remedy. The germ was not the cause of the disease. This led them to develop potentised nosode remedies from these non-lactose fermenting bacilli.

Take the example of *Morgan Bach*, a type of non-lactose organism most frequently found in the stool. The keynote of this remedy is "congestion". It serves well in congestive headaches, mental depression, congestions in gastric mucosa, congestion in the respiratory system, and so on. A study of Japanese patients suffering from dysbiosis confirmed the efficacy of Bowel Nosodes wherein 69.6% patients showed improvements (Tanaka, 2018).

Nearly a century later, Western medicine has tried to ape the homeopathic discoveries with Faecal Microbiota Transplant (FMT). In this process faecal bacteria and other microbes from a healthy individual are transferred into another individual. Faecal microbiota transplant is approximately 85–90% effective in people with *Clostridioides Difficile Infection* (CDI) for whom antibiotics have not worked or in whom the disease recurs following antibiotics. Most people with CDI recover with one FMT treatment (Bakken, et al., 2011).

However, FMT comes with risks, something that potentised Bowel Nosodes do not suffer from. FDA has informed health care providers and patients of the potential risk of serious or life-threatening infections with the use of FMT. The FDA is now aware of infections caused by enteropathogenic *Escherichia coli* (EPEC) and *Shigatoxin*-producing *Escherichia coli* (STEC) that have occurred following investigational use of FMT that it suspects are due to transmission of these pathogenic organisms from FMT product supplied by a stool bank company based in the United States (US Food & Drug Administration, 2020).

Homeopathic bowel nosodes by contrast are free from such risks.

Fast-forward to Covid-19 times

A study was conducted to compare gut microbiome diversity and composition in SARS-CoV-2 PCR-positive patients whose symptoms ranged from asymptomatic to severe versus PCR-negative exposed controls. Patients were classified as being asymptomatic or having mild, moderate or severe symptoms based on National Institute of Health criteria. Exposed controls were individuals with prolonged or repeated close contact with patients with SARS-CoV-2 infection or their samples, for example, household members of patients or frontline healthcare workers. Microbiome diversity and composition were compared between patients and exposed controls at all taxonomic levels (Hazan, et al., 2022).

It was possible to hypothesise that low bacterial diversity and depletion of *Bifidobacterium* genera either before or after infection led to reduced pro-immune function, thereby allowing SARS-CoV-2 infection to become symptomatic. This dysbiosis pattern is a susceptibility marker for symptomatic severity from SARS-CoV-2 infection and may be amenable to pre-infection, intra-infection or postinfection intervention (Hazan, et al., 2022).

It is remarkable that these findings already existed in Homeopathic literature nearly a hundred yeas ago.

Mind is the Key

It has been found that specific emotions play an important role in disease. But is it possible to predict future disease by studying emotions wrought by life-changing events? "Life changes" cover a broad range of events – from matters relating to occupation, residence, community, family, marriage, and the like. It has been found the more these life-changes accumulate in a person's life, the more is the likelihood of experiencing a major illness within the following year (Rahe, 1968).

Studies have indicated that there is a specific relation between the attitude that a person develops towards life and the disease or symptoms he/she develops in response to it. By attitude is meant the combination of two things, namely, (a) what a person feels is happening to him/her, and (b) what he/she wants to do about it, i.e., what action he/she wishes to take. It is assumed that different physiological processes underly each disease, then by extension, each attitude is associated with its own specific set of physiological changes (Graham, Stern, & Winokur, 1958).

One study in 1962 found 18 attitudes predicted certain specific illnesses. For example, it was found that urticaria was associated with the feeling that the person was, "taking a beating and was helpless to do anything about it". Similarly, in the case of acne it was found that the underlying mental state was that of *"being frustrated, feeling blocked of being unable to make oneself understood"*. Low backache was associated with the *"desire to run away or walk out of there"* (Graham, et al., 1962).

While these findings are a big step in finding the association between an illness and the emotional states, it does little by way of finding a suitable remedy. Current Western model of medicine finds no use for such information. Other than an academic interest, it has little to offer in terms of a remedy or cure.

Once again, homeopathy is miles ahead. As we have seen earlier, every remedy undergoes a Homeopathic Pathogenetic Trial (HPT), which is conducted on healthy persons to elicit symptoms in accordance with the Law of Similars. Subsequently, the remedy is used in the clinic to confirm its action on persons in sickness. For each of the examples given above, a suitable remedy can be found.

Bach Flower Remedies Therapy

Dr. Edward Bach was referred to earlier in connection with the development of Bowel Nosodes. Bach was an allopathic doctor and surgeon who later became a bacteriologist and studied homeopathy. Homeopathy made a deep impression on him, and through his spiritual practices he concluded that mental and emotional states held the key not only to wellness but were also associated with certain remedies. Dr. Edward Bach went one step ahead. He discovered remedies prepared from flowers that could be associated with a basic human emotion. The process of preparing the remedies is extremely simple (albeit sensitive) and anyone can prepare them provided some simple steps are followed.

This book will not discuss these remedies in detail but suffice to say that this therapy is yet another example of the theme of this chapter which is *Future in the Past*. What was discovered and put into clinical practice by Dr. Edward Bach in the 1920s and 1930s, has been rediscovered recently by research on stress and disease. It has demonstrated the important role emotions play as a causative factor in disease. For example, anger contributes to pathophysiology of cardiovascular disease. In terms of specificity, specific emotions such as, anger, sadness, embarrassment can be linked with particular health outcomes such as, cardiovascular disease, musculoskeletal disease, etc. (Levenson, 2019).

CHAPTER 7

Fragmentation of Medical Science

"Human science fragments everything in order to understand it, kills everything in order to examine it."

– Leo Tolstoy, War & Peace

Fragmentation of Medical Science refers to the present trend of division and specialization of medical fields. This is supposedly done for a more comprehensive understanding and treatment of various medical conditions. It allows doctors and researchers to specialize in a particular area of medicine. But has it necessarily resulted in greater expertise, efficiency, and improved patient care?

The reality is that it has led to a lack of communication between different medical specialties, and this has divided it into multiple, often conflicting, schools of thought or ideologies. All this has led to gaps in treatment and diagnosis, followed by confusion and difficulty in making informed medical decisions. For example, in the United States, healthcare system is facing enormous problems of unsustainable cost increases, poor quality, and inequalities (Stange, 2009). Because the healthcare system is fragmented and lacks an integral value chain, the only way forward lies in collaboration and an integrated care approach.

This is quite ironical, because today we have more research findings and more technology available than ever before, yet healthcare is not getting any better. Therefore, many feel that the only way forward is to promote interdisciplinary collaboration and communication among healthcare professionals. This is because for the increasingly large number of people with one or more chronic disorders, a more "generalist" approach is needed. The modern system of education of health professionals follows the biomedical model and reinforces fragmentation through the development of specializations and sub-specializations or super-specializations. The primary goal of this system is to create a professional who will serve the system well (Detsky, Gauthier,SR, & Fuchs, 2012). This is why patients are often (or mostly) given the least priority in the education system.

Failure of Reductionist and disease-specific approaches

As a result of this fragmentation, medical science has been reduced to a reductionist, disease-specific approach. In this approach, the human being is a collection of cells, organs and diseases. What is forgotten is that disease means dysfunction of the entire being, and not a malfunction with a group of cells or organs. It is sad that healthcare has now become disease-care and the doctors have been reduced to being mere technicians who are repairing the body. In short, the fragmentation of medical science has led to situation where the patient has become redundant in the system. Healthcare has been reduced to a commodity and health professionals are service providers and patients are consumers.

In recent times, the development of expensive diagnostic devices and immunological drugs has diverted attention from the need for the development of comprehensive geriatric and palliative care. This has led to a focus on specific procedures or services rather than on comprehensive and integrated care. It seems that the direct beneficiaries of this system are not patients, but professionals. Once upon a time, a doctor used to visit patients with his doctor's bag. Today's doctors need a rich healthcare ecosystem to be truly what they were trained for!

Food as medicine

Hippocrates (5th century BCE), the ancient Greek philosopher and physician had famously said, *"If you want to learn about the health of a population, look at the air they breathe, the water they drink, and the places where they live"*.

Any student of medical history will be quick to grasp that most of the health successes in the last 150 years has been possible because of better standards of sanitation, hygiene, nutrition and housing – and all these have been achieved largely through political means that integrated medicine, social development, and poverty alleviation. However, in medical education across the world, very little attention is paid to nutrition and public health. This is very obvious if we review the syllabus of the MBBS course at India's top medical school – the All India Institute of Medical Sciences (AIIMS, 2005).

A 2021 survey of medical schools in the U.S. and U.K., published in the Journal of Human Nutrition and Dietetics, found that most students receive an average of just 11 hours of nutrition training throughout an entire medical program (Millard, 2023). The present state of nutrition education in medical courses is pathetic, to say the least. The present medical model of treatment is only based on pharmacology and surgery. Thus, medical students learn about vitamin C and how it impacts various pathways in the body, as well as what deficiency might look like. These things are indeed important, but doctors struggle to relate this to patient care in terms of what to eat and what not to eat! Doctors find it challenging to translate their learning which is hyper-focused on nutrients to the real-life questions a patient may have about food.

Contrast this with Homeopathy. Back in late 1700s and early 1800s, long before the role of vitamins, minerals and nutrients were discovered, Dr. Samuel Hahnemann, the founder of homeopathy, the importance of nutrition was emphasised as mentioned in Aphorism 77 of the sixth edition of the *Organon of the Medical Art* (Hahnemann, 2013). Hahnemann stressed on the fact that the importance of individualization in nutrition, taking into account a person's unique health status, symptoms, and constitution. Today, homoeopathic nutrition following Hahnemann's guidelines is still followed by practitioners and is considered a complementary approach to medicine.

Some of the key principles of homoeopathic nutrition include the use of foods, herbs, and nutrients that have been shown to have healing properties, as well as avoiding highly processed foods. It is now possible to correlate appetite for some particular foods with body's needs. We have an in-built mechanism in our body that guides us in the matter of quality and quantity of food we need. This is the reason why symptoms relating to appetite, cravings and aversions form such an important part in homeopathic case-taking and analysis. For example, aversion to old cheese is specific to *China officinalis* whereas, a strong desire for goat cheese is characteristic of *Samarium sulphuricum* (which incidentally has also been used by practitioners in cases of rheumatoid arthritis).

In homoeopathy, each remedy has a particular food relation. Some examples of these relations are given below:

For the remedy *Aconite napellus*, food such as alcohol, beer, butter and fatty foods, pork, sour and acidic foods must be avoided. The recommended foods are coffee, cold drinks and milk. Likewise, for the remedy *Lycopodium clavatum*, foods that need to be avoided are beans, alcohol, dry foods, eggs, fatty food, fish, flatulent food, milk, oysters, shellfish, sweets, wine. The recommended foods are hot food, warm drinks, and warm food. Similarly, for the remedy *Hepar sulphuris* foods that need to be avoided are alcohol, brandy, butter, cold drinks, cold water, fatty food, sour and acidic foods. The recommended foods are spices, and highly seasoned food (Rehman, 2004).

This concept of combining nutrition and dietary regimen is unique to homeopathy as it defines diet and regimen on the basis of the individual patient, the disease and the remedy. The subtle interaction of these three elements are best illustrated in the footnote to Aphorism 259 of the Organon, *"The gentlest notes of a distant flute in the still of the night, which would raise a soft heart to over-earthly feelings and melt it away into religious rapture, become inaudible and futile amid the extraneous clamour and noise of the day"* (Hahnemann, 2013).

Frustrations of a doctor

The frustrations of doctors arise from the crisis of the medical profession - the foundations on which it rested for decades, that is, the monopoly of knowledge, autonomy, and self-regulation have been shaken. The emergence of *"Doctor Google"* and other AI-led digital technologies have strongly changed the asymmetry of knowledge, and thus the roles of power and the status of doctors in society. So modern medicine is firmly trapped by many unrealistic expectations and unused opportunities. Thus, today doctors do not have exclusivity in illness and health - a state of affairs that represents a change in the decades-old paradigm (Džakula, Vočanec, & Lončarek, 2023).

CHAPTER 8

They Dared to Be Different

"If you want things to be different, perhaps the answer is to become different yourself."

– Norman Vincent Peale

As we have seen in the previous chapters, modern medicine has increasingly become fragmented, dissociated from patient care, and with overmedication has led to death due to iatrogenesis. A growing chorus of discontent suggests that the once-revered doctor-patient relationship is on the verge of collapse. Public distrust in the pharmaceutical industry has increased, in part due to perceptions of pharmaceutical manufacturers as profit seekers, and in part due to their actions such as off-label marketing, overcharging, and concealing data. Approximately 60% of individuals at high risk for cardiovascular disease did not trust pharmaceutical manufacturers. Lack of trust was higher among those in poor health or without a usual source of care, raising concerns that vulnerable populations have experiences where trust has been broken (Singh, Eisenberg, & Sood, 2023).

In such circumstances we find many allopaths have switched over to homeopathy. In this chapter we shall see three examples of allopaths who undertook this transformative journey.

Dr. A.U. Ramakrishnan

Dr. A.U. Ramakrishnan trained in allopathic medicine in India at the prestigious Madras Medical College and graduated in 1966. He lost a sister and a brother to cancer. Both were medical doctors and that led him to explore farther. He trained in homeopathy at the Royal London Homeopathic Hospital under Dr. Margery Grace Blackie (1898-1981), the first woman Royal Physician to Queen Elizabeth II. Since then, he has been teaching, practicing and conducting post-graduate courses in India, East Asia, Western Europe and North America.

The personal tragedies he suffered led him to focus on cancer. He went on to develop his own methodology trying different combinations, potencies, and dosages of remedies in the treatment of cancer. From late 1980s he began to see favourable responses and over the next few years he experimented with new techniques of prescribing. Dr. Ramakrishnan found that homeopathy is so vast and multifaceted in its healing action that it encompasses a number of distinct approaches in its methodology. Every practitioner has a unique style and can approach the illness by different methods. Dr. Ramakrishnan discovered that the classical approach of a single remedy, single dose of remedy matching the totality of symptoms and the constitution of the patient was not effective against cancer (Ramakrishnan & Coulter, 2001).

According to Dr. Ramakrishnan, in acute ailments and highly specific types of illness (e.g., chickenpox, influenza, etc.) a limited number of medicines appear to work best, regardless of the constitution or personality and mental outlook of the patient. The same applies to cancer. Because of the severity and in many cases urgency of the condition, the individuality of the patient must yield to the specificity of the disease itself. In the treatment of cancer one is dealing with a measurable pathology and not with subtle imbalances of the energies of the body.

In the treatment of cancer, the doctor cannot "wait-and-watch". A more aggressive approach is required.

The treatment protocol developed by Dr. Ramakrishnan can be summed up as, (1) frequent administration of the remedy on a "regulated" basis, (2) prescribing a second remedy in alternation with the first on a regular (usually weekly) basis, (3) administering the remedy by a special method developed by him, and (4) employing a *split-dose-method*.

Dr. Ramakrishnan uses one of two cancer nosodes *Carcinosin* and *Scirrhinum* and alternates these with wide-spectrum cancer-specific remedies and organ-specific remedies. The former are principally *Conium, Thuja,* and *Arsenicum album*. Besides, as mentioned above, there are around 21 organ-specific remedies.

The rates of success of the treatment methodology speak for themselves. Given below is a snapshot comparing pre-1993 and post-1993 (the year he adopted his unique method). It should be noted that a case is considered "successful" must have a five-year non-recurrence rate. It is a fact that many patients turn to homeopathy in the last stages of cancer after they have exhausted traditional Western treatment procedures. Hence, success rate is based on *viable* cases only.

1. Brain cancer: success rate improved from 37% to 70%.
2. Oral cavity cancer: success rate improved from 69% to 86%.
3. Larynx and vocal cord cancer: success rate improved from 46% to 70%.
4. Thyroid and parotid cancer: success rate improved from 58% to 71%.
5. Oesophagus cancer: success rate improved from 53 to 80%.
6. Mediastinal cancer: success rate improved from 33% to 73%.
7. Breast cancer: success rate improved from 57% to 80%.
8. Lung cancer: success rate improved from 29% to 58%.
9. Stomach cancer: success rate improved from 35% to 55%.

10. Pancreatic cancer: success rate improved from 40% to 75%.
11. Liver cancer: success rate improved from 14% to 32%.
12. Colon cancer: success rate improved from 33% to 40%.
13. Rectum cancer: success rate improved from 69% to 82%.
14. Bladder cancer: success rate improved from 56% to 72%.
15. Ovarian cancer: success rate improved from 55% to 69%.
16. Cervical cancer: success rate improved from 38% to 68%.

The list goes on, and I would encourage readers to read the books by Dr. Ramakrishnan.

Dr. Ramakrishnan does not discount *constitutional* treatment – his observation is that is follows his protocol once the cancer is healed. Also, he finds homeopathy is highly effective in conjunction with a number of Western medical procedures. So, a patient stands to benefit best if the oncologist is willing to cooperate and work with a homeopath.

Dr. Jaswant Patil

Dr. Jaswant Patil graduated with an MBBS degree from the prestigious Grant Medical College, Mumbai. He went on to complete his MD in Chest specialisation from Seth G S Medical College, KEM Hospital, Mumbai. For twelve years, Dr. Jaswant Patil worked as a physician in Chest Medicine, General Medicine, Cardiology, Haematology, intensive care and as a House Physician in numerous reputed institutions such as Jaslok Hospital. He was very successful in his field and treated thousands of patients during his allopathic days. Like other allopathic doctors globally, Dr. Jaswant Patil also negated the success of homeopathy treatments and could not bear the sight of his patients taking homeopathy pills.

Sadly, around 1993, Dr. Patil's mother fell seriously ill and suffered from multiple organ failure with septic shock. All the intensive care treatment were of no avail and her condition was rapidly getting worse. At this point he recalled that when he was a student studying for his MD degree, he had been suffering from chronic pain which was cured by homeopathy.

Out of curiosity he had bought a few books on homeopathy, but soon lost all interest. Given the condition of his mother, out of sheer desperation, Dr. Patil decided to give homeopathy a chance. To his astonishment, his mother recovered in just two days! That was the watershed event that brought Dr. Jaswant Patil into the fold of homeopathy.

Dr. Patil went on to complete the Bachelor's program in Homeopathy (BHMS) and later expanded his horizon and has integrated many other "alternative" therapies in his practice. He has seen over 100,000 patients. He has designed a unique non-invasive Cardiac Rehabilitation Program which is exclusively available at his centre.

Dr. Surjit Singh Makkar

The first homeopath to arrive in India was Dr. John Martin Honigberger who hailed from Transylvania in Romania. He was a contemporary of Dr. Samuel Hahnemann. He arrived in Lahore, the capital of the Sikh empire in the Punjab and was presented at the court of Maharaja Ranjit Singh. He impressed the Maharaja by treating his favourite horse who was suffering from bad ulcers of the leg. Thus, the first spectacular successful case of homeopathic treatment in India was a veterinary case!

Dr. Surjit Singh Makkar also hails from the Punjab and is a veterinarian doctor. He chose to cross-over to homeopathy. Dr. Surjit Singh began his career as a veterinarian doctor in the government of Punjab Animal Husbandry department. Early in his career a poor farmer brough his buffalo who was suffering from mastitis to the clinic. Dr. Surjit Singh prescribed the standard set of drugs – penicillin and steroids. The farmer reported that the udder we no longer swollen, the redness had subsided and there was no discharge from the teats. The farmer however returned a few weeks later and was virtually in tears. His buffalo has stopped giving milk. The allopathic treatment that followed did not help. Dr. Surjit Singh was deeply moved by the plight of the poor man. He had probably pledged his wife's jewellery to buy the buffalo and he said that feeding a buffalo with no yield would only make him poorer. Dr. Surjit began a study of Ayurvedic and homeopathic literature. He found a rich repertoire of homeopathic remedies to address agalactia in milch animals. He collated all the symptoms and observations and the most suited remedy appeared to be *Phytolacca decandra*. He gave the buffalo the remedy and the buffalo recovered very fast. This was a momentous revelation. Dr. Surjit thereafter adopted the use of homeopathic remedies in all his veterinary cases.

Quite early in his practice Dr. Surjit realised that in India there were not many books on veterinary homeopathy. Also, there was a need to develop an easy-to-use computer program to help veterinarians to deal with cases in day-to-day practice. So, he pursued a Masters in Information Technology (MSc IT) and Masters in Computer Applications (MCA) and developed his own software.

Dr. Surjit Singh feels homeopathy has a major role to play in veterinary medicine. A treatment which would normally cost a dairy farmer in India ₹ 5,000 (US$ 60) by using allopathic medicines can be treated more effectively, with no adverse effects, and in a shorter period of time with homeopathic medicines for just ₹ 100 (US$ 1.20)! Homeopathy has a larger role to play in the village economy of India. Healthier animals with higher yield bring in more prosperity and wellbeing of the entire village community. He heels homeopathy has a major social and economic role to play in the progress of every nation. To help the layperson Dr. Surjit Singh has a helpline, an online quick-reference guide for common ailments. He has published over 35 research papers in various international journals and was conferred the *Rastriya Gaurav* Award for meritorious services, outstanding performance and remarkable role in veterinary homeopathy by the India International Friendship Society.

Thus, we can see how homeopathy transformed the outlook of Dr. Surjit Singh, a formal veterinarian and in effect transformed society around him.

Dr. Aadil Chimthanawala

A young cardiology post-grad intern at a leading hospital in Nagpur, India reported on duty. As he was about to enter the Intensive Coronary Care Unit, he noticed a man in his thirties pacing up and down the war corridor frantically. He seemed unwell. He approached him and the man extended his hand, not so much for a handshake but as a hand extended for help. When the young doctor held his hand around the wrist, and he instinctively felt his pulse. He found he was really suffering from arrhythmia and was very anxious. He told the doctor that his mother had been just admitted to the ICCU. The doctor assured him she was in very competent hands and that he should not really worry. The man said he was not doubting the capability of doctors but was worried that he was not capable of meeting the medical expenses in case his mother had to undergo any surgery. The young doctor understood the son's worry and his cause of panic. He felt helpless too. He entered the ICCU and checked the charts of the mother. It looked grim. She was not stabilizing and no clear line of treatment had been planned.

The doctor's father was a reputed homeopath, so he called him on the phone and sought his advice. His father prescribed *Aconitum ferox*. The doctor arranged for the remedy and gave a dose to the mother. The mother started responding. Over the course of the next few hours, and changing remedies to match the symptoms, the lady condition stabilized, and she was moved to the general ward. The patient's family was in tears. Not only had a life been saved, but they had also been saved from a possible financial ruin. It was a turning point in the life of the young cardiologist too.

The young cardiologist is Dr. Aadil Chimthanawala. He comes from a family of doctors and his father Dr. Karim Chimthanawala too is an allopath who turned to homeopathy. From an early age he had seen patients flock to his father's clinic, but he also wanted to be cardiologist. He had always held an impeccable academic record and was also adjudged the Best Cadet in National Cadet Corps. So, taking up admission in the MBBS course seemed to be an obvious choice. He topped the pre-medical entrance exam and graduated in 1998. He completed his post-graduation in cardiology specialty and the incident narrated above happened. He immediately decided to study homeopathy and instead of pursuing a lucrative professional practice enrolled for the BHMS course at the Nagpur College of Homeopathy and Hospital.

Dr. Aadil has been practicing homeopathy since. He specializes in cardiology cases and true to the Hahnemannian dictum serves his patients with homeopathic remedies, dietary regimen, exercise, and lifestyle changes. But his contribution to society is not restricted to clinical practice. The National Academy of Homeopathy India founded by him has "adopted" two villages to provide free medical care. He began by running OPD camps every week or fortnight. Patients came out of curiosity and also because it was free. One day a patient asked the doctor if he had a cure for his cow who was suffering from mastitis. Dr. Aadil gave him a remedy and in the next visit he found the patient count had doubled – thanks to the cow who had recovered almost immediately!

At this stage the village folk asked him if he could help them with growth problems of their farm plants. He prescribed *Silicea* to improve the plants' ability to thrive. Not only the plants thrived but also developed resistance to fungal and pest attacks! This won their trust and faith in homeopathy. Dr. Aadil found that village communities are more informal, personal and their crops, plants and animals form part of their community. Therefore, instead of holding camps he distributed remedy kits with basic remedies and simple instructions for their use. That went a long way in empowering and binding a community.

This experience gave Dr. Aadil a new direction in his community work. He had been organising courses and seminars for students and practitioners of homeopathy. He started making short 5-minute videos on common ailments and remedies to educate the general public – laypersons, housewives, and mothers. His YouTube channel has nearly 500 videos, 12,000 subscribers and a million views.

Thus Dr. Aadil has increased the scope of homeopathy from being a mere medical intervention into a community building tool. People whose lives are rich in social capital naturally cope better with traumas and more effectively fight illness. Social bonds work better than vitamin C, antacids, and sleeping pills.

CHAPTER 9

First Do No Harm

"Primum non nocere" (First, do no harm).

– Hippocrates of Chios (460 BCE – 370 BCE)

Primum non nocere is a Latin phrase that means "first, do no harm." It is often associated with the 4th century BCE Greek physician Hippocrates of Chios who is attributed to have introduced it as an oath to swear to never intentionally harm a patient. In modern times, the phrase has come to symbolize the importance of avoiding unintended consequences in scientific research and medical treatments. However, in today's practice, most doctors think it is an albatross around their neck because there is hardly any treatment, they offer which is without harm (Lecroy, 2001). Strangely they overlook the fact that homeopathic treatment never provokes adverse effects (Dantas & Rampes, Do homeopathic medicines provoke adverse effects? A systematic review, 2000).

Iatrogenesis

Iatrogenesis is the causation of a disease, a harmful complication, or other ill-effect by any medical activity, including diagnosis, intervention, error, or negligence. This can include errors in administration, adverse drugs reactions, surgical complications, and medical devices. In a study of 815 consecutive patients on a general medical service of a university hospital, it was found that 36 percent had an iatrogenic illness (Steel, Gertman, Crescenzi, & Anderson, 2004). Some iatrogenic events are obvious, like amputation of the wrong limb, while others, like drug interactions can evade recognition. Iatrogenesis can include mental suffering via medical beliefs or a practitioner's statements.

The causative factors include adverse effects of prescribed drugs or vaccines, overuse of drugs or adverse interactions between prescribed drugs. Medical error is a term that is narrower in definition and refers to misdiagnosis, incorrect prescription, faulty procedures, or plain negligence. As reported by Johns Hopkins Medicine, it is now accepted that medical error is the third leading cause of death in the United States, and 10 percent of all U.S. deaths are now due to medical error (Daniel, 2016). Another study concludes that a significant proportion of hospitalization-associated disability of elderly hospitalized patients may be induced by iatrogenic events, and that most of them are potentially preventable (Sourdet, et al., 2015). In fact, depression, infection, disability, dysfunction, and other specific iatrogenic diseases now cause more suffering than all accidents from traffic or industry (Illich, 1974).

Iatrogenesis is not limited or restricted to physical injury done to patients by ineffective, toxic or unsafe treatments. It has a social and a cultural dimension too. Social iatrogenesis results from the medicalisation of life. More and more of life's problems are seen as amenable to medical intervention. Pharmaceutical companies develop expensive treatments for non-diseases. Cultural iatrogenesis refers to the destruction of traditional ways of dealing with and making sense of death, pain, and sickness. As Illich describes, "Society, acting through the medical system, decides when and after what indignities and mutilations the patient shall die." This is particularly of concern because modern medicine has led to increased longevity with more opportunity to accumulate chronic diseases.

Overmedicalization and overdiagnosis

Ivan Illich was a theologian, philosopher, sociologist, and historian. He was a was a radical thinker who rallied against the system of standardized health care, and he coined the words *iatrogenesis* and *overmedicalization*. He had famously said that the major threat to health in the world today is modern medicine itself, and he was referring to *overmedicalization*. A well-established example of increasing medicalisation for childbirth is caesarean section rates. In a span of just 15 years five European countries, the Slovak Republic, Czech Republic, Ireland, Austria and Hungary more than doubled their caesarean delivery rates (Declercq, Young, Cabral, & Ecker, 2011).

Overdiagnosis can be defined as the detection of abnormalities that are not destined to ever bother us or that will never cause symptoms or death. One way is to cultivate "thought leaders" who "raise awareness" through campaigns which seek to transform the "worried well" into the "worried sick".

An example of overdiagnosis the treatment of hypertension. Firstly, this condition is nothing more than a diagnosis based on a cut-off point. In the end, this diagnosis solely serves to identify a risk factor for cardiovascular conditions, such as heart attack and stroke. Secondly, in the focus on lowering this risk with pharmaceutical treatment we may overlook that hypertension is one of several risk factors, and, even more important, can be lowered or prevented with lifestyle change.18 By looking at hypertension from a purely medical view, other risk factors such as an unhealthy diet, obesity, and physical inactivity are easily overlooked.

Another example of misdirected overdiagnosis that is well documented is mammography screening. Even after 20–30 years of mammography screening, the incidence rates of advanced and metastatic breast cancer have remained stable, in other words, no improvements have emerged.

Breast cancer mortality rates have not decreased more rapidly in areas where mammography is in place since the late 1980s. What is alarming is that one third (33%) to one half (50%) of mammography-detected breast cancers would not have been clinical during lifetime - a classical textbook example of overdiagnosis. In other words, the role of mammography screening in reducing breast cancer is much debated. These findings are based on a meta-analysis of numerous studies in Western European countries (Autier & Boniol, 2018).

In the year 2017, a panel of surgeons in India has called on professional surgical societies to tackle the twin problems of unethical surgical practices in the private healthcare sector. They appealed to surgical societies to make efforts to reduce "healthcare corruption" in private hospitals. A Mumbai based medical second opinion services centre has found an uncomfortable truth. Almost 44% of the patients for whom surgery was recommended were advised against it in their second opinion. Here is a newspaper report which is quoted below.

Take the case of Kandivili resident Gaurav Sharma whose uncle was advised cardiac surgery due to severe left shoulder pain. "We were told to undergo cardiac surgery the next day itself. Our entire family went into a tizz wondering what to do". He logged into MediAngels' online chat with a cardiac surgeon in Delhi who looked at the ECG and said the patient only had an orthopaedic problem. "I then sought the opinion of a shoulder specialist based in the US. He diagnosed that my uncles shoulder and arm bones were not aligned properly. He showed my uncle some shoulder exercises on an aonline chat", said Sharma and added that his uncle's pain reduced significantly (Iyer, 2015).

Hysterectomy, the surgical removal of the uterus, is the most common non-obstetric gynaecological surgery amongst women in the reproductive age group, according to the Federation of Obstetric and Gynaecological Societies of India (FOGSI) and Integrated Health and Wellness Council report. The most common medical indications for hysterectomy include fibroids, abnormal uterine bleeding, uterine prolapse, chronic pelvic pain and premalignant and malignant tumours of uterus and cervix. In India, hysterectomies are the second most common gynaecological surgery, often conducted for conditions like heavy menstrual bleeding (HMB), which could be managed non-surgically (Dutta, 2023). According to a Thomson Reuters report, 95% of the hysterectomies carried out in the private sector hospitals are unnecessary.

Among the unethical practices followed by many doctors in India, are, prescribing more tests than necessary - to be done at preferred labs, keeping you admitted at hospital rooms when you're fit to be discharged, prescribing expensive medicines/vaccines when cheaper and quality substitutes are available, charging patients at different rates for the same treatment, fake operations as described above, forcing pregnant women to undergo C-section when it is not required, and last but not the least, luring poor, uneducated people to donate organs, kidney in particular, for which there is no dearth of high paying patients.

Another unethical practice is the "racket" of referrals. Many doctors are lured or scared into paying commissions to other doctors in return for having patients referred to them. The current rate of such commissions, is between 40% and 60%, which means that if a patient paid Rs 1,000 to the doctor reffred to, he will have to pay between Rs 400 and Rs 600 to the doctor who referred the patient to him (Vora, 2017).

Homeopathy – a welcome contrast

Homeopathy is not driven by nor is subservient to the pharmaceutical companies or the insurance companies. The data for all remedies is available in the public domain in the form of published materia medica. The *provings* of any remedy can be replicated and confirmed clinically (Reilly, et al., 1994). Also, numerous studies and meta-analyses have confirmed that homeopathic remedies do not produce any adverse effects (Dantas, et al., 2007).

CHAPTER 10

Magic of the Minimum Dose

"What is there that is not poison? All things are poison, and nothing is without poison. Solely the dose determines that a thing is not a poison".

– Paracelsus (1493-1543)

Swiss-born Paracelsus is considered the "father of chemistry and the reformer of materia medica," and had been given the epithets such as the "Luther of Medicine," the "Godfather of modern chemotherapy," the "founder of medicinal chemistry", and the "founder of modern toxicology". Paracelsus and his followers espoused the position that like cures like; that is, "a poison in the body would be cured by a similar poison," (principle of similitude) but the dosage is very important. Although he wrote that "nature hints at cures," he felt that many medicinal preparations lacked sufficient "potency" to treat current diseases (Borzelleca, 2000). However, he was never able to find a workable solution which could be put into clinical practice.

The principal issues of iatrogenesis and overmedication raised by Ivan Illich are only addressed adequately by homeopathy, which is essentially based on individualization, use of a minimum dose of high dilution, potentized remedies. The principle of the minimum dose was also observed by Arndt-Schultz who enunciated the fundamental principles of Neurosomatic Therapy. What Arndt-Shultz discovered was that weak stimuli excite physiological activity, moderate stimuli favour it, and strong stimuli arrest it. In other words, stimulus beyond the optimal dose will lead to weakening or absence of the effect. The dose–response relationship is a central concept in many biological disciplines, but especially in pharmacology, toxicology, and risk assessment. Sadly, despite its centrality in the biological sciences, the origins of dose–response concepts and models remain underexplored and underappreciated in allopathy.

A "working hypothesis" for homeopathic effects seems to be that, during the potentization process, "information" or "energy" is being preserved or even enhanced in homeopathic remedies. The organism is said to be able to pick up this information, which in turn will stimulate the organism into a self-healing response.

Dr. Samuel Hahnemann was the first physician who tested the tenets of Paracelsus and discovered the Law of Similars described in an earlier chapter. When Hahnemann first announced cures of diseases by extremely small doses of medicine, his statements were received with disbelief and ridicule. Hahnemann's appeal to the medical profession to test the new method and publish results to the world was met by active opposition. He was forbidden to practice and was driven from his home by relentless persecution. Hahnemann had claimed that a dilution as minute as billionth of a grain (dilution ratio of 10^{-9}), could be effective. To orthodox practitioners, who in most cases prescribed drugs by the spoonful, the ideas of Hahnemann were ridiculous. Hahnemann in his defence tried to point out that classical literature from the times of Galen and Paracelsus all supported his claims fell on deaf ears.

Homeopathy is not an indicative method like allopathy in which one medicine treats one disease. Rather it is a system in which remedies are customized to individuals, based on broad themes of constitution, age, and idiosyncratic characteristics identified from the totality of the patient's physical, mental, emotional and pathological symptoms. Each patient will require a series of remedies along the path of cure to match the stages of disease and accompanying symptoms. This means each patient for a "named" disease may require a different remedy.

Complexity science and homeopathy

One of the principal obstacles to homeopathy's general acceptance has been its perceived lack of sound theoretical basis within accepted reductionist, deterministic biophysical medical thought. This could be overcome if we were to look at the nondeterministic concepts of the physical sciences, e.g., quantum theory and its notions of entanglement, nonlocality, and uncertainty. Thus, the concept of Patient-Practitioner-Remedy Entanglement (PPR) explained to in a later chapter, represents a new complementary strand of thought with the potential to create a new theoretical basis for homeopathy.

Totality versus Polypharmacy

Polypharmacy is truly the bane of allopathy causing unnecessary harm. In the past, polypharmacy was referred to the mixing of many drugs in one prescription. Today polypharmacy implies to the prescription of too many medications for an individual patient, with an associated higher risk of adverse drug reactions (ADRs) and interactions. Sadly, polypharmacy is a widespread problem, and physician, clinical pharmacists and patients are all responsible. More than twenty years ago, in 2002 a US survey indicated that 25% of the overall population takes five or more medications per week (Rambhade, Chakarborty, Shrivastava, Patil, & Rambhade, 2012). Polypharmacy may occur when additional drugs are prescribed to treat the adverse effects of other drugs. This is known as the "prescribing cascade". It is sometimes overlooked because the symptoms it causes can be confused with symptoms of normal aging or another disease. Sometimes it results in still more drugs being prescribed to tract the new symptoms.

Case study

Let us now look at a case-study from a standard textbook prescribed in medical colleges the world over. It appears in the first chapter (page 5), titled Introduction to Therapeutics (Ritter, Lewis, Mant, & Ferro, 2008), and is summarised below.

"A GP reviews the medication of an 86-year-old woman. The patient lives in a nursing home, has hypertension and multi-infarct dementia. Earlier her family used to visit her, but now she no longer recognises them. She needed help in dressing-up, washing, and feeding. When the GP examined her he found she smelled of urine, and had several bruises on her head, although she seemed well-cared for. She was calm, but pale and bewildered.

"Her rectum was loaded with hard stool. Her pulse was 48 beats per minute, and her blood pressure lying down was 169/96 mmHg, and 122/76 mmHg while standing. She was sweating and distressed while standing. Her urine sample was sent for analysis and the culture showed only light mixed growth.

"The GP stopped all medications, and a manual evacuation of faeces was performed. The stool was found negative for occult blood, and her full blood count was normal.

"Two weeks later, she was incontinent only at night, and was normal during daytime. Her heart rate was now 76 beats per minute and her BP while lying and standing was 208/108 mmHg. The following drugs which were prescribed prior to stopping all medication seemed to be causing the following conditions:

   i. *Postural hypotension due to Imipramine, Bendroflumethiazide, Haloperidol*
   ii. *Constipation due to Imipramine, Haloperidol*
  iii. *Reduced mobility due to Haloperidol*
   iv. *Constipation due to Haloperidol*

 v. *Bradycardia due to Atenolol*
 vi. *Urinary incontinence due to Bendroflumethiazide*
 vii. *Aspirin could have caused GI tract bleeding at a later stage."*

The lesson learnt is that drugs for prevention do not help after the event. More importantly, polypharmacy can cause tremendous harm and suffering.

Totality

Homeopathy, by contrast, does not prescribe different medicines for different symptoms but addresses the condition of the patient on the basis of "totality". Totality goes beyond just the numerical total of physical signs and symptoms. In fact, the treatment of multimorbid patients who have a combination of three or more concurrent complaints is one of the core competencies of homeopathy. There are numerous approaches of determining the totality of symptoms for determining the remedy.

The concept of totality takes into account, (i) the seat of the disease, (ii) the cause, (iii) changes in temperament brought about by the disease, (iv) any peculiarities which are not explained by the disease, (v) modalities, i.e., what makes the patient feel better or worse, and (vi) any concomitant symptoms.

This is best illustrated by a case-study.

A man aged 35, reported (i) pain in the right deltoid region, (ii) following an embarrassment in an office meeting. (iii) He was sleepless at night due to pain and (iv) any movement made it feel worse, (v) and he felt better after sunset, typically between six to 9 pm. (vi) The pain seemed to radiate downwards along the arm. (vii) He also reported that he used to get palpitations in his heart anytime he was anxious.

At first sight this would appear to present very sketchy set of physical symptoms, that are primarily subjective, but potentially serious, and cannot be quantified by diagnostic tests. A physician would order an

ECG, ask for a neurological examination, and prescribe pain killers, sleeping tablets, and anti-anxiety drugs. These drugs would in turn cause their desirable and not-so-desirable symptoms.

A classical homeopath would use each of those symptoms to find a single matching remedy. Usually, the homeopath would use a computerised software to analyse. In the instant case there is just one single remedy, namely, *Kalmia latifolia* that covers all the symptoms. He was administered a single dose of the remedy, to be repeated once a day. Two weeks later, he reported no pain, and undisturbed sleep. He felt less anxious and felt no palpitations.

This case is not unique. It occurs in everyday practice of every homeopath.

We must remember that polypharmacy is an increasing concern. The global prevalence, especially amongst the elderly, is around 62% (Zhao, Chen, Xu, Fan, & Tian, 2023).

CHAPTER 11

Homeopathy: Beyond the Disease Model

"The good physician treats the disease; the great physician treats the patient who has the disease."

– Sir William Osler, MD

The critics of homeopathy admit that homeopathy is remarkably popular, and in the same breath allege that the assumptions underlying homeopathy violate fundamental laws of nature. Or, it is argued that homeopathy does not have any explanatory power and fails other criteria established for a scientific approach. However, according to the United Nations' World Health Organisation homeopathy is the second most popular system of medicine. In India, where homoeopathy is a national medical system, the market is growing at 25% a year, and more than 100 million people depend solely on this form of therapy for their health care. India has almost a quarter of a million registered homeopathic doctors – more than any other country in the world. So, what sets homeopathy apart?

Disease versus illness

Disease and illness are two different though interrelated concepts. This distinction though is often overlooked. While disease defines a pathophysiologic process, illness is defined by the state of the complete person—physical, psychological, social, and cultural. Patients suffer illness while doctors diagnose and treat disease. Illness is an experience, while disease in the medical model is an abnormality in function or structure of body parts or organs. The boundaries between health and disease, between well and sick, are far from clear and never will be clear, for they are diffused by cultural, social, and psychological considerations. In lighter vein, Dr. Eric J. Cassell had said, illness is "what the patient feels when he goes to the doctor", and disease is "what he has on the way home from the doctor's office.

Diseases are the named pathological entities that makeup the medical model of ill-health, such as diabetes or tuberculosis, and which can be specifically identified and described by reference to certain biological, chemical or other evidence. Thus, diseases are seen as abstract "things" or independent entities which have specific properties and a recurring identity in whichever setting they appear (Helman, 1981).

Most cases of disease are accompanied by illness because illness is a psychological, cultural and the cultural reaction to the disease process. In some cases, disease can occur in the absence of illness. This subtle distinction is often missed by the allopath but is appreciated by the homeopath. For example, in some cases of asymptomatic hypertension or early stages of cancer, patients may be told they have a named disease but there is no experience of illness. Likewise, illness can also occur in the absence of disease. Hypochondriasis is one example. Subjective feelings of not feeling well which are often of psychological origin and for which no physical cause can be found. A doctor who only emphasises on the treatment of disease, without considering the illness dimension, may be indifferent to a patient in whom no physical disease is found.

A bio-psycho-social model of health

The Biopsychosocial (BPS) model of health was conceptualised by George Engel in 1977. He suggested that to understand a person's medical condition it is not simply the biological factors one has to consider, but also the psychological and social factors (Engel, 1977).

It is a useful model for primary care or family doctors. Sadly, even though 40 years have passed since Engel introduced this concept, there is still minimal use of the biopsychosocial model in education, clinical care, and research dominated by allopathy. It is now accepted that disease onset, especially for non-communicable diseases, also known as the long-term conditions (LTCs), has a complex, multifactorial causation, involving many risk factors of relatively small effect, affecting multiple and often diverse outcomes.

Homeopathy – *future in the present*

What is overlooked is the fact that homeopathy has been using a model like the BPS model for the past 250 years! The homeopath views the patient as a unit of organic, mental, and social dimensions of life. This contrasts with the biophysical view of health which is essentially reductionist. In 1790, Immanuel Kant made the famous statement, *"There will never be a Newton of the blade of grass, because human science will never be able to explain how a living being can originate from inanimate matter"* (Schuster, 2011). That holds true even after more than two centuries.

A homeopath takes into account a complete picture of the patient in order to understand the suffering of the patient and then finds a remedy that suits the condition. To understand this concept, let us examine a case. This case is presented by Dr. Heiner Frei in his book on polarity analysis, a classical technique of homeopathic case analysis (Frei, 2013).

"Mr. F comes to the emergency clinic. After a winter walk the previous day, he had severe, acute, shooting pains in the left lower jaw and left cheek, with twitching of the entire left side of his face. The pain comes in fits lasting around 30 seconds. An accompanying symptom is nosebleeds (bright red blood). At the same time, the patient feels the familiar premature ventricular contractions (PVCs) more intensely and more frequently than before. He has been having these for the past ten

years, but not in this way. He is anxious because he has been taking anticoagulants for a prior heart attack although he nevertheless suffered a deep-vein thrombosis in the leg two years ago."

The interview with the patient reveals the following subjective symptoms:

"He feels worse during sleep. Symptoms are aggravated in general by cold and drafts of air but feels better when wrapped up. He is worse when touched or by application of pressure on the affected area."

A homeopath would consider the subjective symptoms as more important as they describe the person in disease rather than the disease in a person. The symptoms that make a person feel better or worse are called modalities. Analysis of these modalities would point to three or four principal remedies. Dr. Heiner Frei found that *Rhus Toxicodendron, Belladonna, Arnica* and, *Bryonia* scored the highest. *Belladonna* was selected because it covers violent neuralgia, twitching of facial muscles, convulsive movement of facial muscles, shooting and tension of lower jaw, and tearing/drawing behind right zygoma. All these symptoms are observed in the provings of the remedy *Belladonna* (Allen T. , 2021).

The aftermath:

"Mr. F. is given a dose of Belladonna 200C. He phones the next day to say that he had a good night. He calls again the following day to say that the trigeminal neuralgia has completely disappeared, and he can no longer feel the PVCs. No relapse over an observational period of 10 years."

The annals of homeopathy medical literature are full of such cases, one only needs to have an open mind. As Paracelsus had said, *"The Art of Healing comes from nature, not from the physician. Therefore, the physician must start from nature, with an open mind"*. If we open our minds to the possibility, there is always more to learn.

CHAPTER 12

Homeopathic Hospitals – The Way Forward

"Homeopathy is a progressive and an aggressive step in medicine."

– John D. Rockefeller

Patients – the new victims of corporate hospitals

Recently, the Chief Justice of India, NV Ramana while addressing the National Academy of Medical Sciences said there has been a growing distrust in the common citizens towards doctors and hospitals, and "hefty fees, chaotic experiences, and sub-par service has marred the relationship between doctors and the general public". He went on to say that the profit driven approach of hospitals denies the poor access to healthcare (Choudhary, 2022).

Privatisation of the National Health Service in the UK is real and is showing the effects of decline. Private firms were handed GBP 15 billion (US\$ 19 billion), and the government used the Covid-19 pandemic to transfer NHS duties to the private sector, even though overwhelmingly 84% of the people tend to prefer a 'publicly run' health service. (Nuffield Trust, 2020). What are the implications of this? How do quality of care and patient outcomes change after private equity acquisition of hospitals?

In a paper published in the prestigious Journal of the American Medical Association (JAMA), it has been reported that on average, private equity acquisition of hospitals was associated with increased hospital-acquired adverse events. This study covered 662,095 hospitalisations at 51 private equity-acquired hospitals and 4,160,720 hospitalisations at 259 control hospitals between 2009 and 2019. There was a 25% increase in hospital-acquired conditions, surgical site infections doubled from 10.8% to 21.6% despite a reduction of 8.1% in surgical volume.

The decline and demise of homeopathic hospitals in the West are a direct consequence of the machinations of the hospital industry.

Once upon a time, there was the Royal London Homeopathic Hospital which was founded in 1849. Frederic Foster-Quinn, the first homeopathic physician in England, had been instrumental in the founding it. Gradually the support from the government declined. In the year 2010 it was renamed the Royal London Hospital for Integrated Medicine and thereafter in the year 2018 ceased offering homeopathy. The fate of the Bristol Homeopathic Hospital, founded in 1832 closed in 2015. The Liverpool Homeopathic Hospital which opened in 1887 closed shop in 1976, and so did the Tunbridge Wells Homeopathic Hospital, which was founded in 1902, shut shop in 2009.

Just how much was the government actually spending to justify shutting down these homeopathic hospitals? In the British House of Commons Science and Technology Committee Report of 2009-2010, Mr. Mike O'Brien, Minister for Health Services gave oral evidence, *"In terms of drugs it is £152,000 a year which comes from a budget of £11 billion. It is approximately 0.001 percent, we calculated, of the drugs budget"* (House of Commons, 2010). Isn't that preposterous? Or is starving the funding a part of larger pharmaceutical industry driven agenda?

Homeopathic hospitals – India experience

Homeopathy is very popular in India. India leads in terms of the number of people using homeopathy, with 100 million people depending solely on homeopathy for their medical care, and the market is growing at 25%

a year (Prasad, 2007). One reason homeopathy has thrived in India is due to people's belief in the holistic approach to health, which takes into account the physical, emotional, and mental well-being of an individual. Additionally, the use of natural, non-toxic remedies is also appealing to many people. Further, the country's rich cultural history and diverse medical traditions have allowed for the integration and adaptation of homeopathy into Indian medicine.

India is unique because it has recognised homoeopathy as an official and legitimate system of medicine and has given it the status of a national medical system at par with allopathy and Ayurveda. Homeopathy enjoys the support of the Government in India. In 1973, the government set up the Central Council of Homeopathy (CCH) to regulate its education and practice. There are over 250,000 registered homeopathic doctors currently, with approximately 12,000 more being added every year Homeopathy has blended well into the roots and traditions of the country. Seven out of ten diseases recognised as a national health burden are the most commonly reported diseases at the homeopathy wellness centres in India. Homeopathy units comprise 1/19th of the number of allopathy units, yet the annual patient footfall in the former is 1/5th of the latter (Kaur, Chalia, & Manchanda, 2019). By contrast, homeopathy in the USA has been in steep decline from the 1920s.

As mentioned earlier, homeopathy is insulated against the machinations of the hospital system and pharmaceutical industry largely because it is not negatively impacted by the development or regulation of drugs, potentially for financial or other motives. Indeed, valid criticism of the pharmaceutical industry often snowballs into demonization, and that is what we must avoid.

There are numerous government-run homeopathic hospitals in every state in India. Most large hospitals have a homeopathic facility attached. All homeopathic colleges offering the Bachelor's programme have a homeopathic hospital attached to the institute. Also, there are many private homeopathic hospitals too, and the services provided are exemplary.

Case-study: Aditya Homeopathic Hospital – Pune, India

One shining example is a private hospital purely dedicated to homeopathic cure. It is located in Pimpri village in Pune district of Maharashtra State. Aditya Homeopathic Hospital and Healing Centre was founded and conceived by Dr. Amarsinha Nikam, a third-generation doctor. Dr. Nikam was motivated by his desire to help the poor with affordable healthcare. He had a strong background in treating acute cases and dealing with emergencies in remote rural areas with homeopathy alone. Most people could not imagine that a hospital providing only homeopathic care would be a viable project. He began with a four-bed setup in 1995, and today it is a 100-bed hospital with an out-patient department that runs 24 X 7 throughout the year. It has a well-equipped ICU and uses state-of-the-art diagnostic tools. The hospital attracts many interns from all over the country as they wish to learn homeopathic practice in a hospital setting. Additionally, the hospital provides training and conducts many seminars.

Dr. Nikam felt the necessity of opening a homeopathic hospital because even if mainstream hospitals have homeopathic consultants in their OPDs, they are not available all the time. Even private practitioners work during fixed hours and "pull their shutters down" and go home at the end of their busy day. A full-fledged homeopathic hospital alone can give 24 X 7 X 365 care to patients. His hospital deals with every type of case, be it acute pericarditis, cardiac myopathy, endocarditis, myocardial infarction, acute renal failure, acute appendicitis – every conceivable condition that would require immediate medical attention and admission to a hospital. The hospital deals with Multiple Sclerosis, trigeminal neuralgia, psoriasis, brain tumours and many such conditions for which a patient may not find much help in a General Hospital or a

Specialty Unit. Aditya Homeopathic Hospital has an ambulance so that patients do not lose time reaching us. So far more than 3,000 critical cardiac cases have been successfully treated here. As Dr. Nikam tells us, "In all cases we have demonstrated the efficacy of homeopathy not only on the basis of a 'feel good' sensation reported by the patient, but also with the support of diagnostic tests and clinical parameters."

In days gone by, doctors used to watch the patients or get regular nurse practitioner reports on the patients who monitored the day and night. Today, at Dr. Nikam's hospital patients are monitored on CCTV to understand symptoms, modalities and peculiarities that may not be evident in a case-taking session.

Nowadays people are having a crisis of confidence with regard to the medical field. Modern medicine has earned a bad name because of the suffering and financial exploitation borne by patients. Homeopathy is more relevant today than ever before because it does no harm, it is a gentle way to cure, the cure goes to the root of the disease, and is very affordable. Patients admitted to the General Ward in the hospital pay just Rs. 300 per day (less than US\$ 4/ GB£ 3), including the cost of medicines.

The secret of success of Dr. Nikam's practice is that he follows the classical style of homeopathic practice that prescribes a single remedy in a single potency, does not use any combination remedies or patented mixtures, and case-management is fully transparent. That is how a homeopathic hospital can remain free from the clutches of the pharmaceutical corporations. As Dr. Nikam says, even Hahnemann (the founder of Homeopathy) was an allopathic doctor and homeopathy was born out of his desire to reform the system as it existed during his time. Hahnemann's words are as relevant today as they were in the 18th Century. Homeopathy is not based on conjecture, theory, or logic. It is based on understanding the Dynamic Laws of Nature, on observations during *provings* and on experience in the clinic. The human mind constantly seeks patterns where none exist, whereas remedy proving and the experience in the clinic are unbiased observations (RajGuru, 2015).

It is well known that drug companies resist prescription of generic drugs and encourage, through incentives and coercion, the use of branded drugs. For example, patients are prescribed Tylenol instead of acetaminophen which is functionally the same. Drug companies pay drug reps - to promote familiarity with a drug and its brand name. And because brand names are more expensive, they have a significant burden on the health care system (Hansen, 2018). On an average, a generic drug is between 80% to 85% cheaper than the branded equivalent. Based on a study of over one million prescriptions over a four year period found that for certain drugs, the brand name was used overwhelmingly more than the generic— in some cases, by nearly 100 to 1 (Ouyang, Tisdale, Ashley, Chi, & Chen, 2018). This was so despite the fact that on an average, acetaminophen received a rating of 6.2 out of 10 with only 29% reporting negative effects, against Tylenol received a lower rating of 5.9 out of 10 with as many as 33% reporting negative effects (Drugs,com, n.d.).

This goes to show how homeopathic practice steers clear of branded drugs and all prescriptions are essentially generic – they are derived from *provings* as explained elsewhere in the book.

CHAPTER 13

The Strawman Arguments Against Homeopathy

"The scientific method is not a test for truth, but only a means of determining the probability that a particular theory is correct."

– Alfred Wegener

Alfred Wegener was a German meteorologist and a polar explorer. A hundred years ago he first proposed that the continents had once been massed together in a single supercontinent (which he named Pangaea), and then gradually drifted apart. He was widely ridiculed and soon mostly forgotten. Geologists thought that continents stood anchored firmly on a solid earth and were permanent features. At a Royal Geographical Society meeting, an audience member thanked the speaker for having blown Wegener's theory to bits! But, in the mid-1960s, as older geologists died off, and younger ones began to accumulate proof of seafloor spreading and vast tectonic plates grinding across one another deep within the earth. They came up with the now accepted theory of tectonic plates, which *explains* what Wegener had proposed.

Compare this with the following remarks made by Nobel laureate Venkatraman Ramakrishnan, who said, *"They (homoeopaths) take arsenic compounds and dilute it to such an extent that just a molecule is left. It will not make any effect on you. Your tap water has more arsenic.*

No one in chemistry believes in homoeopathy. It works because of the placebo effect" (Thakur, 2016). It is quite surprising that such a statement comes from a Nobel laureate, and it raises the question of whether one calls something wrong if it cannot be explained by our current knowledge of natural phenomena. As we saw above, Wegener was ridiculed just because geologists and others had not gathered the wherewithal to observe seismic activity, plate motions, crustal deformation, and the presence of rocks, minerals, and other crucial inputs.

Let us look at the record of homeopathy, which is quite similar to the case of Wegener.

Emil Adolf von Behring won the first Nobel Prize in medicine or physiology for his discovery of the diphtheria antitoxin. Later, he discovered the tetanus antitoxin. In 1892 Behring actually experimented with serial homeopathic dilutions and found paradoxically enhanced immunogenic activity. But he was advised to suppress this experiment due to the aid and comfort it would provide to homeopaths! Only after he won the Nobel Prize did he feel comfortable in making public these experiments (Behring, 1905).

Popular narratives to decry homeopathy

Allopathy rejects seemingly solid evidence because it is not compatible with a theory they support. But that is not unusual. They also do the same within conventional medical science - sometimes they discard a theory because of new facts, but at other times they cling to a theory despite the facts! Indeed, many arguments seem logical at first sight but turn out to be fallacious on closer inspection.

Homeopathic remedies are prepared from medicinal substances through a series of dilutions and rapid shaking (succussions) or trituration between the dilutions. As the level of dilutions increases progressively, the remedy gets more *potentized*. The main argument against homeopathy is that these series of dilutions soon reach a limit whereby even a single molecule of the original substance does not exist in the preparation. As a result, it is concluded that homeopathy does not adhere to contemporary chemical principles, thereby making any claim about its effects pharmacologically implausible. Indeed, homeopathy presents a "new language", and critics are unwilling to learn it. Therefore, the doors are already closed at the beginning of the debate, and for them, homeopathy simply has no right to exist.

The main characteristic of science is that all knowledge is provisional. And the only argument against homeopathy is ultra-dilution of remedies.

Countering the strawman arguments

There is no reason to believe that the influence of publication bias, data massage, bad methodology, and so on is much less in conventional medicine, and, as mentioned earlier in this book, the financial interests for regular pharmaceutical companies are many times greater.

Are the results of randomised double-blind trials convincing only if there is a plausible mechanism of action? Are review articles of the clinical evidence only convincing if there is a plausible mechanism of action? Or is this a special case because the mechanisms are unknown or implausible? For example, take the case of Alzheimer's disease. For years, the prevailing theory has been that Alzheimer's is caused by pileups of proteins called amyloids, which effectively create plaques in the brain. But drugs that help clear amyloids from the brain don't seem to work very well in combating the disease.

Without getting into an example of life sciences and the attendant complexities, let us consider a simple phenomenon that physics has not been fully able to explain, and yet we use it in everyday life – flying in an airplane.

We take airplanes for granted. The total number of passengers flown by air globally in 2019 was approximately 4.5 billion. It is the safest mode of travel. Yet, shockingly, as reported by the prestigious journal *Scientific American*, no one can explain why airplanes stay in the air! Science, in its present state, has not been able to solve the mysteries of aerodynamic lift! (Regis, 2020).

Another more shocking example is that of our knowledge of the force of gravity. In the words of Richard Panek, a Guggenheim Fellow in science writing, and the author of *The Trouble with Gravity: Solving the Mystery Beneath Our Feet*, "Nobody knows what gravity is, and almost nobody knows that nobody knows what gravity is. The exception is scientists. They know that nobody knows what gravity is, because they know that they don't know what gravity is." (Panek, 2019). In simple language, science has not been able to satisfactorily explain why gravity exists, but that does not prevent us from making pendulum clocks, using a siphon in our toilet flush tanks, or building hydroelectric turbines to generate electricity, or children sliding down a ramp or enjoying on the see-saw! So, Panek asks to contemplate on the question, is gravity just a word, or a semantic convenience or a mere "placeholder" till a better noun comes along?

In the case of hormone replacement therapy (HRT), the best evidence has caused the medical approach to change overnight, even if it contradicts the theory. HRT was started in the 1960s, with very high popularity in the 1990s. The first clinical trials on HRT and chronic postmenopausal conditions were started in the USA in the late 1990s. The first results of the Women's Health Initiative in 2002, showed that HRT had more detrimental than beneficial effects (Cagnacci & Venier, 2019).

Need to clean the Augean Stables

There are several instances of fraud and dishonesty in academics and clinical medicine. But at the root of it is not mere lust for lucre, it is often sponsored and supported by the most prestigious and revered institutions. There are many forces at work, and these are driven by market forces, the medical establishment and an academic logic. One such case is that involving the Karolinska Institutet, in Sweden, the most prestigious institute in Sweeden, and a star surgeon Paolo Macchiarini.

Macchiarini had pioneered transplant operations of artificial windpipes embedded with stem cells. This was based on two papers that described the procedure. These papers had not received the necessary ethical approval, and that a seventh paper also authored by Macchiarini, reporting transplantation of artificial oesophagi into rats, had misrepresented results, too. Macchiarini's research had been hailed as a bright spot in the field of regenerative medicine, which has been frustratingly slow to deliver on its promise of allowing synthetic materials to act as replacements for natural organs. His procedure involved bathing a specially made polymer tube shaped like a trachea in stem cells taken from the transplant-recipient's bone marrow. The idea was that when this was transplanted to replace a damaged trachea, the cells would form the necessary type of tissue and create a seal with the surrounding tissue (Cyranoski, 2015).

Indeed, Macchiarini's procedures sound very scientific and sound in theory, but in reality were a monumental failure that caused many deaths, agony and suffering to patients and their families. What is more appalling is the fact that Macchiarini stated that it was never his responsibility to obtain any necessary permissions he was not directed to do so, nor did he have the authority to do so. So much for good science from the institution that is responsible for selecting the Nobel Prize laureates in physiology or medicine. Macchiarini was sentenced to a prison term of 30 months by a court in Sweden, but strangely, Karolinska Institute was let off the hook despite the fact that this misconduct happened right under its nose. This is a shameful contrast to homeopathy which allegedly fails the test of being supported by a viable scientific theory.

The fact that modern science is not able to explain how and why homeopathy works, should not be a valid reason for dismissing it as pseudo-science. It is unethical, unscientific, and truly unbecoming for a Nobel laureate like Venkatraman Ramakrishnan to denigrate homeopathy. It only displays arrogance and ignorance.

Possible cause of bigotry against Homeopathy

I have always wondered why Homeopathy, which originated in the West, is facing such difficult times in that culture (although Germany is an exception – there is no legal monopoly on the practice of medicine). If you follow debates broadcast over the media in the US and the UK (and now Australia), you will find the views against Homeopathy virtually stink of bigotry. By contrast, Homeopathy is accepted and respected in places like India, Malaysia, Sri Lanka and in most South American countries.

Is there a deeper reason for such attitudes?

One view presented by some medical anthropologists is that present day practice of biomedicine in the West has evolved in a culture dominated by monotheistic traditions of belief. Monotheism is founded on a commitment to "universal truths", and "unitary paradigms". This has nurtured a culture of allowing only a single-minded approach to illness and care [9]. In the countries mentioned above, the medical pluralism matches the social and religious pluralism seen in society. One will find that medicine, like religion, ethnicity and other key social institutions, is a medium through which the pluralities of social life are expressed and recreated (Klienman, 1995).

However, institutionalized modern medical practice in these pluralistic societies is also a victim to the same "medical monotheism" of the West. Thus, it will not brook an alternative concept like Homeopathy. By contrast, ethnomedicine systems, be they TCM or Ayurveda, are open to ideas, concepts and practices of modern science and work towards a synergistic relationship. In these countries practitioners of all hues will often send their patients to a Homeopath (and vice-versa) for a difficult and chronic problem which has no clear-cut cure in their system.

One of the outgrowths of this has been that the institutions of Allopathy have complete control over establishing the criteria by which Homeopathy is judged. Another area of difference that lies in the world view of Allopathy is its insistence on questioning the grounds of knowledge within the present frame of knowledge. If Life Force cannot be measured, weighed or imaged, it is ridiculed to be non-existent. Similarly, therapeutic efficacy is measured only on the basis of RCTs and not by any other method.

But Homeopathy is not the only victim of this social order. Even within the practice of modern medicine, there is a tacitly approved caste system. Psychiatry, internal medicine, paediatrics and the like are viewed as the "soft" side of practice and the real "hard core" medicine is surgery. The "soft" specialties provide low incomes and attract more women practitioners, while the "hard" specialties pay more and command more respect. Perhaps that is one reason why some soft specialties like dermatology (internal medicine) have added surgery to their practices.

Given these realities, where do you think a homeopath giving sugary pills stands in the hierarchy?

The moral of the story is that there are many matters that cannot be presently explained in a scientific way - for instance, physiological and psychological effects of high dilution solutions of homeopathic remedies, but that does not mean they should be treated as unscientific. Perhaps the only one way out is that we may have to wait for some historical singularity – an event which will break the ivory towers of allopathic arrogance, just like communism, caste-system, slavery, imperialism and many more dogmas and practices had their day, only to be swept away by the winds of liberal change.

CHAPTER 14

Evidence in Support of Homeopathy

"The fact that an opinion has been widely held is no evidence whatever that it is not utterly absurd."

– Bertrand Russell

Several renowned epidemiologists have stated that the proof for homeopathy is not inferior to the proof for conventional medicine, even though there are others who merely brush this fact aside and claim it is just a placebo effect. But real-life experience is quite the contrary.

Forty percent of general practitioners in the Netherlands practice homeopathy. In Britain, 42% of general practitioners refer patients to homeopaths. Against this evidence is a backdrop of considerable scientific scepticism!

Testimonials of celebrities

Many celebrities, statesmen, and even doctors have vouchsafed for the efficacy of Homeopathy. Let us look at some examples before we move on to hard evidence.

The best poster boy for the use of homeopathy is King Charles III, the monarch of Great Britain. For three generations the Royals have been depending on homeopathy for primary health care. After his coronation the King appointed seventy-year-old Dr. Michael Dixon as the Head of Medical Household. Dixon trained as a general practitioner and is a Fellow of the Royal College of Physicians, and a Fellow of the Royal College of General Practitioners but is a great supporter of homeopathy. Before studying medicine, he graduated in psychology and philosophy from the University of Oxford. In other words, he has had a well-rounded education and training and is not a quack as newspapers would make you believe. His appointment raised hackles in the mainstream media who called his appointment as a "controversial" decision and claimed that his appointment undermines evidence-based medicine.

In 1932 George Bernard Shaw, a renowned novelist, dramatist and literary critic who was awarded the Nobel Prize for literature, wrote an essay titled *Doctors' Delusions, Crude Criminology and Sham Education*, which included a story about the homeopathic treatment he received for a hydrocele. This accumulation of fluid around the testicle normally requires surgery. Thanks to homeopathy, Shaw experienced a rapid cure without recurrence. Shaw once challenged Sir Almroth Wright, FRS, the noted bacteriologist and immunologist, to look into homeopathy's ability to cure many "incurable" diseases. Wright expressed complete incredulity, while Shaw retorted that Wright had no scientific attitude or simple curiosity (Ullman, 2007).

Dr. Luc Montagnier is a French virologist who won the Nobel Prize in 2008 for discovering the AIDS virus. He surprised the scientific community with his strong support for homeopathic medicine. In an interview published in *Science* magazine of December 24, 2010 he expressed support for homeopathy. Said, *"I can't say that homeopathy is right in everything. What I can say now is that the high dilutions are right. High dilutions of something are not nothing. They are water structures which mimic the original molecules."* (Enserink, 2010). Clearly, Venkatraman Ramakrishnan was not up-to-date in his knowledge and allowed his bias to overshadow his scientific acumen.

There are many other Nobel laureates who supported homeopathy. One good example is Gabriel García Márquez (1927–2015), the Colombian novelist and journalist who won the 1982 Nobel Prize in Literature. In his novel *Love in a Time of Cholera*, the godfather of the novel's protagonist is a homeopathic doctor, and ironically, the protagonist is fighting for the affections of a woman who is married to a conventional physician!

Another Nobel prize winner, Mother Teresa (later beatified as Saint Teresa) studied homeopathic medicine with Dr. Diwan Jai Chand (1887–1961), a highly respected Indian homeopath. According to a report from a conventional physician who worked closely with Mother Teresa from 1945 through at least 1988, the Mother "believes that homeopathic treatment is indispensable for the poor and distressed people of all other countries of the world, for its easy approach, effectiveness, and low cost" (Ullman, 2007).

The great Indian polymath, Rabindranath Tagore, the first non-European to win the Nobel Prize for Literature asserted, *"I have long been an ardent believer in the science of Homeopathy and I feel happy that it has got now a greater hold in India than even in the land of its origin. It is not merely a collection of a few medicines but a real science with a rational philosophy as its base. We require more scientific interest and inquiry into the matter with special stress upon the Indian environment"* (Baghi, 2000).

Other modern-day famous people who have publicly declared their interest in and support for homeopathic medicine include: Catherine Zeta-Jones, Whoopi Goldberg, Pamela Anderson, Jane Fonda, Cher, Rosie O'Donnell, Martin Sheen, the Chili Peppers, Jane Seymour, Lesley Anne Warren, Axl Rose, Linda Gray, Susan Blakely, Michael Franks, Cybill Sheppard, Vidal Sassoon, Angelica Houston, Boris Becker, Martina Navratilova, Priscilla and Lisa Marie Presley, Cliff Robertson,

Jerry Hall, Diane von Furstenberg, Ashley Judd, Naomi Judd, Olivia Newton-John, Julianna Margulies, JD Salinger, Blythe Danner, Pat Riley (coach of the Miami Heat), and England's former Prime Minister Tony Blair.

Other famous people who have been known to use homeopathic medicines: Charles Dickens, W.B. Yeats, William Thackeray, Benjamin Disraeli, Pope Pius X, Louisa May Alcott, Susan B. Anthony, William Lloyd Garrison, Daniel Webster, Harriet Beecher Stowe, Henry Wadsworth Longfellow, William Seward, artist Jackson Pollock, W.C. Fields, and former American Presidents James Garfield and William McKinley.

Data from studies

A few studies are quoted below, and a search on the Google Scholar will show more than 30,000 papers.

1. A meta-analysis of 93 clinical trials of homeopathy showed significant benefit of homeopathy and 41 failed to discern any inter-group differences, and only two described an inferior response with homeopathy (Mathie, 2003).

2. A meta-analysis published in 1991 was designed to establish whether there is evidence of the efficacy of homoeopathy from controlled trials in humans. The results showed a positive trend regardless of the quality of the trial or the variety of homoeopathy used (Kleijnen, Knipschild, & Riet, 1991).

3. Thirty databases/sources were used in another study to identify studies reporting on homeopathy in depression, published between 1982 and 2016. Studies were assessed for their risk of bias, model validity, aspect of homeopathy and comparator. Eighteen studies assessing homeopathy in depression were identified. Two double-blind placebo-controlled trials of homeopathic medicinal products (HMPs) for depression were assessed.

Homeopathy was found to be comparable to antidepressants and superior to placebo in depression, and patients treated by homeopaths report improvement in depression (Viksveen, Fibert, & Relton, 2018).

4. Many cancer patients seek homeopathy as a complementary therapy. A prospective observational study with cancer patients in two differently treated cohorts: one cohort with patients under homeopathic treatment (HG; n = 259), and one cohort with conventionally treated cancer patients (CG; n = 380). For a direct comparison, matched pairs with patients of the same tumour entity and comparable prognosis were to be formed. 120 patients of HG and 206 patients of CG met the criteria for matched-pairs selection. An improvement of quality of life as well as a tendency of fatigue symptoms to decrease in cancer patients under complementary homeopathic treatment was observed (Rostock, et al., 2011).

5. Thirty clinically subjects with Benign Prostate Hypertrophy (BPH) were given individualised homeopathic treatment and followed up for a period of 1 year. Treatment effects were analysed periodically by American Urological Association score (AUA score) and ultrasonography.

   Marked amelioration of symptoms and reduction in size of prostate gland in BPH subjects were observed after homeopathic treatment when analysed by AUA score and ultrasonography. There was marked reduction in various symptoms of BPH such as nocturia, straining, incomplete sensation after urination, interrupted flow of urination with dribbling of urine and urgency significantly from 21.60 ± 4.64 units to 12.23 ± 3.68, that is, ~57% reduction in symptoms of obstruction of bladder problem (Gupta, Singh, & Saxena, 2019).

6. The aim of another study was to determine the possible effect of two homeopathic medicines, ***Ruta graveolens 5CH*** and

Rhus toxicodendron 9CH, in the prevention of aromatase inhibitor (AI) associated joint pain and/or stiffness in women with early, hormone-receptor positive, breast cancer. Aromatase inhibitors are a class of drugs used to treat some forms of cancer.

Women were recruited in two groups, according to which of the two study centres they attended: one receiving homeopathy in addition to standard treatment (group H) and a control group, receiving standard treatment (group C). All women were treated with an AI. In addition, women in group H also took *Ruta graveolens* 5CH and *Rhus toxicodendron* 9CH (5 granules, twice a day) up to 7 days before starting AI treatment. The results suggested that treatment with *Ruta graveolens* 5CH and *Rhus toxicodendron* 9CH may decrease joint pain/stiffness in breast cancer patients treated with AIs (Karp, et al., 2016).

7. A pilot study was undertaken to explore the effect of homeopathic medicines in treating people with non-erosive gastroesophageal reflux disease or non-erosive reflux disease (NERD). People enrolled were having heartburn and/or regurgitation symptoms at least twice a week and having a gastroesophageal reflux disease (GERD) symptom score of more than 4. Significant differences were found in pre- and post-treatment GERD symptom score. Homeopathic medicine was prescribed on the basis of the presenting symptoms. Response to treatment was assessed on GERD symptom score, visual analogue scale (VAS) for heartburn, and the World Health Organization quality of life-BREF (WHO-QOL) questionnaire evaluated at baseline and at the end of 8 weeks of treatment.

   Besides that, statistically significant improvement was also seen in three domains of the WHO-QOL score, i.e. psychological health, social relationship, and environmental domain (Mittal, et al., 2016).

8. A study was conducted to evaluate the benefits of homeopathically prepared *Arnica montana* on post-operative blood loss and seroma production in women undergoing unilateral total mastectomy by administering *Arnica montana* 1000 Korsakovian dilution (1000 K).

   From 2012 to 2014, fifty three women were randomly assigned to *Arnica montana* or placebo and were followed up for 5 days. The main end point was the reduction in blood and serum volumes collected in drainages. Secondary end points were duration of drainage, a self-evaluation of pain, and the presence of bruising or hematomas. The results showed that the use of *Arnica montana* 1000K was associated with a reduced post-operative blood and seroma collection.

9. An Indian research team set out to investigate the effect of individualised homeopathic medicines in improving activity of daily living (ADL) in patients affected by knee osteoarthritis (OA) by reducing pain, stiffness and limiting the disease progress.

   One hundred and thirty one consecutive patients with OA of the knee were recruited and followed up for minimum period of 12 months. Two orthopaedic surgeons diagnosed the disease based on clinical examination of the patients. Three trained homeopathic physicians prescribed individualised homeopathic medicines and the patients were evaluated for pain on WOMAC Osteoarthritis Index LK3.1 (IK) survey form measuring pain, stiffness and ADL. The pain was also measured on numerical pain rating scale (NRS) for further confirmation.

   The homeopathic intervention was associated with a mean ADL score reduction of 35.85 down to 19.08 (p-0.0001). Mean pain on WOMAC Osteoarthritis Index survey form improved from 10.50 to 5.48 (p-0.0001). The mean pain score on NRS improved from 6.34 to 3.77 (p-0.0001) and the mean morning stiffness also improved from 4.55 to 2.18 (p-0.0001) (Motiwala, Kundu, Bagmar, Kakatkar, & Dhole, 2016).

10. Researchers from India's Central Research Institute and Central Council for Research in Homoeopathy compared the effects of individualised homeopathy (IH) with standard allopathic (SA) treatment for people with alcohol dependence using a controlled, open-label design. Subjects were screened verbally using the CAGE scale. 80 people who fulfilled the inclusion criteria were randomised to either IH (n=40) or SA (n=40) treatment and followed up for 12 months.

    The primary outcome was the level of change in the Severity of Alcohol Dependence Questionnaire [SADQ] rating scale at 12 months. Data analysis was done for both intention-to-treat (ITT) and per-protocol (PP) populations.

    The results showed that individualised homeopathy was superior to standard allopathic in the management of alcohol dependence. The medicines most frequently used were *Sulphur*, *Lycopodium clavatum*, *Arsenicum album*, *Nux vomica*, *Phosphorus*, and *Lachesis*.

11. A prospective study looked at the effects of constitutional homeopathy for the prevention of recurrent urinary tract infections (UTI) in patients with spinal cord injury (SCI) in Switzerland. Participants with ≥ 3 UTI/year were treated either with a standardised prophylaxis alone or in combination with homeopathy. The number of UTI, general and specific quality of life (QoL), and satisfaction with homeopathic treatment were assessed prospectively for one year. 35 people were enrolled in the study, with 10 allocated to a control group and 25 received adjunctive homeopathic treatment. The median number of self-reported UTI in the homeopathy group decreased significantly, whereas it remained unchanged in the control group.

The domain incontinence impact of the QoL improved significantly, whereas the general QoL did not change. The satisfaction with homeopathic care was high.

12. Eighty general medical practitioners in Belgium who were physicians and members of the *Unio Homoeopathica Belgica* gathered data about routine homeopathic general practice. A total of 782 patients presented with diseases of all major organ systems which were of sufficient severity to interfere with daily living in 78% of cases.

    Patients reported that compared to previous conventional treatment, though the consultations were much longer they cost less than a third of what allopathic treatment would have. Further, one or more conventional drug treatments were discontinued in over half (52%) of the patients, CNS (including psychotropic) drugs (21%), drugs for respiratory conditions (16%) and antibiotics (16%). The great majority (89%) said that homeopathy had improved their physical condition; 8.5% said that it had made no difference, and only 2.4% said that homeopathy had worsened their condition (Wassenhoven & Ives, 2004).

13. Following a multiple-casualty construction disaster in Israel, members of The Centre of Integrated Complementary Medicine joined in the emergency activity of the Shaare Zedek Medical Center. They administered homeopathic treatment to injured patients to supplement conventional orthopaedic treatment. This was perhaps the first time that homeopathy was used officially in conjunction with conventional medicine in an emergency situation.

    Fifteen orthopaedic patients were included. They were treated by homeopathy in two phases starting 24 hours post-trauma. All patients initially received *Arnica montana* 200CH in a single dose. Anxiety was treated with *Aconite* 200CH in nine patients,

Opium 200CH in three, *Ignatia* 200CH in two and *Arsenicum album* 200CH in one according to type of anxiety. One day later, most patients reported a lessening of pain, 58% felt improvement, 89% had reduced anxiety, and overall, 61% felt that homeopathic treatment was helpful. In the second phase, 48-hour post-trauma, specific complaints were addressed with classical homeopathy. At discharge patients rated the homeopathic treatment successful in 67% of the specific complaints (Oberbaum, Schreiber, Rosenthal, & Itzchaki, 2003).

It is hoped that this will spark sufficient interest in the mind of the reader to explore further. The reader must understand that homeopathy is founded on empirical principles and present-day science is yet not equipped to understand or explain the phenomenon. The conceptual models and the experimental findings from complexity science may support the paradoxical claims of Law of Similars and the potentizing effects of dilution and dynamization through succussion and trituration.

Some of the greatest teachers in medicine, including those from the allopathic practice were quick to understand the underlying complexity of life sciences and medicine. I would like to quote from Harrington's *Principles of Internal Medicine*, a standard text in all medical curricula – *"The practice of medicine combines both science and art. One must be able to identify the crucial elements in a complex history and physical examination. The combination of medical knowledge, intuition, and judgment defines the Art of Medicine, which is as necessary to the practice of medicine as is a sound scientific base."* (Braunwald, et al., 2000).

Conclusion

Indeed, there is a need for viable hypotheses of homeopathy mechanism of action. One of the earliest systematic reviews of homeopathic clinical trials concludes: *"… The amount of positive evidence even among the best studies came as a surprise to us. Based on this evidence we would readily accept that homeopathy can be efficacious, if only the mechanism of action were more plausible."* (Bellavite, Ortolani, Pontarollo, Pitari, & Conforti, 2007).

CHAPTER 15

Plants, Animals, and Soil Bust the Placebo Myth

"The art of medicine consists of amusing the patient while nature cures the disease."

– Voltaire

Placebos, by definition, are "inert substances which can't do anything". Yet it's clear that after the administration of such drugs, things do happen! One of the most common theories is that the placebo effect is due to a person's expectations. If a person expects a pill to do something, then it's possible that the body's own chemistry can cause effects similar to what a medication might have caused.

It is a commonly held belief that homeopathy is 'nothing more than a placebo effect', a turn of phrase which seems to dismiss homeopathy as ineffective. Sadly, such statements also eliminate the role of the placebo in healing. However, experts confirm that the placebo effect is *a real neurobiological phenomenon and that the brain's "inner pharmacy" is a critical determinant for the occurrence of psychobiological and behavioural changes relevant to healing processes and wellbeing'* (Meissner, 2011).

According to the National Health Service (NHS) of UK website, *"Homeopathy is a 'treatment' based on the use of highly diluted substances, which practitioners claim can cause the body to heal itself. A 2010 House of Commons Science and Technology Committee report on homeopathy said that homeopathic remedies perform no better than placebos (dummy treatments)".* For this reason alone, NHS stopped funding homeopathy since 2017 (NHS, 2021).

Detractors of homeopathy turn a blind eye to the fact that for many subjectively experienced conditions, such as pain and depression, rather large placebo effects have been reported. In fact, there is increasing evidence that placebo interventions also affect end-organ functions regulated by the autonomic nervous system. Indeed, an anatomical framework of the autonomic system exists which allopathy sympathisers and homeopathy-bashers seem to be ignorant or turn a blind eye purposefully. It has also been shown that the placebo effect is not limited to subjective psychological feelings alone. This is borne out by the fact that many physiological effects such as such as gastric motility and lung function, improved in placebo-treated patients when compared with untreated controls (Hróbjartsson & & Gøtzsche, 2010)!

More than "positive thinking"

Placebo effect is more than mere positive thinking though. A Harvard university publication confirms that the mind can be a powerful healing tool - when given the chance. The idea that our brain can convince our body that a fake treatment is the real thing has now been confirmed by studies and that under the "right circumstances" a placebo can be just as effective as traditional medical treatments.

Will a person react positively to a treatment where the medication is clearly labelled as "placebo? A study led by Kaptchuk and published in *Science Translational Medicine* explored this by testing how people reacted to migraine pain medication. One group took a migraine drug labelled with the drug's name, another took a placebo labelled "placebo" and a third group took nothing. The researchers discovered that the placebo was 50% as effective as the real drug to reduce pain after a migraine attack. (Harvard Medical School, 2021). That is why engaging in the rituals of "healthy living" — eating right, exercising, yoga, quality social time, meditating — probably provides some of the key ingredients of a placebo effect.

It is now being suggested that a placebo might in fact offer the theoretical advantage of an inexpensive treatment that would not cause adverse drug reactions or interactions with other medications, potentially avoiding complications of polypharmacy (Cherniack, 2010). Indeed, the detection of a significant difference between the therapeutic effects of an active pharmacological agent or procedure and a matched inert placebo has become a challenge for medicine. That is so because factors that contribute to placebo responses have received scant attention.

Cancer-related fatigue (CRF) is a common and challenging late effect for many cancer survivors. Clinical trials prove robust placebo effects on CRF in blinded trials. Clinical trials demonstrated a robust placebo effect on CRF in blinded trials. It was found that that even when administered openly, placebos improved CRF in cancer survivors (i.e., patients knew they were receiving a placebo) (Zhou, et al., 2019).

Can there be a placebo effect in surgery?

A placebo in surgery is a fake surgical intervention that looks like a therapeutic intervention but omits the key step. It's also called sham surgery. It is a faked surgical intervention that omits the step thought to be therapeutically necessary.

In the 1940s and '50s, doctors thought they had found an amazing new way to treat the chest pain caused by a shortage of blood flow to the heart. They cut into patients' chests and tied up two of their arteries. But in 1959, a landmark study put the procedure to the test. In the placebo group, sedated patients got the incisions but no knotted arteries. The results were shocking. Patients who got the sham surgery fared no worse than those who got the actual intervention (Cobb, Thomas, Dillard, Merndino, & Bruce, 1959).

According to a 2014 review, about three-quarters of sham-controlled studies show some improvement. A review found that 72% of studies reported improvement in both the surgical and placebo groups, and 51% reported superiority of the placebo over the surgical procedure (Wartolowska, et al., 2014).

Placebo and the mind – a limited viewpoint

If homeopathy is just a placebo effect and the placebo effect is tied to the workings of the human mind, then certainly, then the placebo effect should not be demonstrable in studies conducted on plants. What is often forgotten is that Homoeopathy is a universal medicine – it works for plants, animals, humans and even soil since it is based on the Law of Similars.

According to a leading newspaper, increasingly farmers are using homeopathy to improve crop and plant health and increase productivity. For more than a decade, the Sri Aurobindo Society has been on the trail of the possible applications of homeopathy in agriculture. After years of research, the Society has started field level experiments in Puducherry and neighbouring states and is working with more than 30 farmers (TOI, 2023).

Homeopathic medicines are used on crops, plants, trees and soil to "cure" diseases and are seen as an alternative to use of chemical fertilizers, fungicides and pesticides in agriculture. Agro-homeopathy also avoids environmental pollution and pesticide toxicity. The cost involved in using this method in agriculture is much lower than in conventional farming. It has scope across the globe if the research undertaken can establish concrete trends in examining the effectiveness of agro-homeopathy not only in increasing the yield but also in its contribution towards controlling pests, retaining the soil health and being safe for the ecosystem.

Neurobiologists have tried to link the placebo effect to neurophysiology. For example, the brain regions involved in the placebo effects on pain and their potential functions in this context have been mapped. These areas include the medial thalamus, anterior insula, dorsal anterior cingulate cortex, periaqueductal and secondary somatosensory cortex-dorsal posterior insula (Wager & Atlas, 2015). How do we explain the positive effects of homeopathy on plants and soil?

In short, placebo effects are beneficial effects that are attributable to the brain–mind responses to the context in which a treatment is delivered rather than to the specific actions of the drug. Further, these effects are mediated by diverse processes including learning, expectations, and social cognition. In other words, placebo responses occur across diverse clinical disorders and are related to objective pathology and survival too. Studies so far have concentrated on determining how placebo treatments affect various health-related behavioural, autonomic, endocrine, and immune measures. How will we relate these discoveries to plants and soil who have no discernible autonomic, endocrine and immune systems, nor do they have identifiable parts of the brain mentioned by Wager and Atlas?

This means, we cannot apply the neurobiological model of explaining the placebo effect outside the realm of human beings, and such explanations are not complete. Thus, explaining homeopathy as mere "placebo effect" is a churlish attempt of the medical establishment in its failure to explain observed phenomena.

All in the plant's "mind"?

The use of agrochemicals like growth hormones, fertilisers, fungicides and germicides has generated numerous negative ecological effects.

Therefore, application of homeopathy to agriculture provides the most obvious alternative.

The studies that have been conducted can be classified into two categories. These are (1) germination and growth models, and, (2) plant pathological assays and field assays. In recent years there is an increase of research in areas of disease control as well as studies of metabolic processes in plants treated with homeopathy. Let us examine a few studies on application of homeopathy to plants.

1. Control of pathogens. In India, Khanna and Chandra obtained significant results in rot control of tomato, caused by *Fusarium roseum*, with the application of homeopathic preparations of *Kali iodatum* in 149CH and *Thuja occidentalis* in 7CH, in pre- and post-harvest conditions. These authors evaluated the quality, palatability of fruits treated and cost of the treatment, concluding that there was practical and economic feasibility in the homeopathic treatment, besides the prophylactic and curative actions. Later on, these same authors, obtained significant results in the control of rot in mango, guava and tomato fruits by the application of various homeopathic drugs in pre and post-harvest conditions, with suppression of spore germination and respiration of the fungi *Alternaria alternata, Colletotrichum gloeosporioides*, Fusarium roseum and *Gloeosporium psidii* (Khanna & Chandra, 1976).

2. Inhibition of fungi. Singh and Sinha, in India tested various homeopathic drugs, and verified that Sulphur (200CH) inhibited 100% the growth of *Aspergillus parasiticus.* The *Silicea terrea* and the *Dulcamara* reduced the growing of the fungi in 50% and the production of toxin in more than 90%. The *Phosphorus* had little effect in inhibiting the growing of the fungi (less than 10%) but reduced it in almost 30% the production of aflatoxins.

3. Reduction of powdery mildew of tomato. Homeopathic drugs act in biological processes of plants without producing toxicity. Rolim and his colleagues demonstrated a reduction of powdery mildew of tomato by using the remedy *Kali iodatum* 100CH, in greenhouse, and increase in number of leaflets by biotherapy obtained from the pathogen *Oidium lycopersici* (Toledo, Stangarlin, & Bonato, 2011).

4. Growth rates of mercury stressed duckweed. Research was conducted to determine whether there is convincing evidence for specific effects of ultra-high dilutions of homeopathic remedies in the case of severely mercury-stressed duckweed (*Lemna gibba L.*). Duckweed was moderately stressed with 2.5 mg/L mercury(II) chloride for 48 hours. Afterwards plants grew in either *Mercurius corrosivus* in (seven different potency levels, 24X–30X), or water controls (unsuccussed or succussed water) for 7 days. Growth rates of the frond (leaf) area were determined using a computerised image-analysis system for day 0–3 and 3–7. Three independent experiments with potentised *Mercurius corrosivus* and three systematic negative control experiments were performed. All experiments were randomised and blinded. Unsuccussed and succussed water did not significantly differ in their effects on duckweed growth rate. The study yielded evidence of growth-enhancing specific effects of *Mercurius corrosivus* 24x–30x in the second observation period (day 3–7), (Jäger, Würtenberger, & Baumgartner, 2021).

5. *In-vitro* studies against fungus *Aspergillus niger*. A study was undertaken with the aim to explore the antimicrobial effect of different homeopathic drugs and its potencies against *Aspergillus niger*, a fungus that is commonly found in soil and decaying plant material. It can cause infections in people with weakened immune systems. Marked antifungal activity was observed with mother tincture of *Zingiber officinale*; the growth of *Aspergillus niger* was inhibited and showed maximum zone of inhibition up to 15.4 ± 2.88 mm followed by *Holarrhena antidysenterica* (13.2 ± 1.09) and *Terminalia chebula* (10.6 ± 1.14). Different potencies (3x, 6x and 12x) were also exhibited significant zone of inhibition, especially *Allium cepa* 6x, *Caesalpinia* *bonducella* 6x and 12, *Eucalyptus globulus* 12x, *Ruta graveolens* 12x, *Thuja occidentalis* 6x, and *Zingiber officinale* 3x and 6x as compared to control (Prajapati, Mahima, & Kumar, 2019).

6. Soil microbial activity. Andrade observed responses on soil microbial activity, by changes on the rhythm of breathing, when applied with homeopathic drugs, demonstrating that these drugs interfere directly in the biomass of soil and, consequently, in the health of the plants (Toledo, Stangarlin, & Bonato, 2011).

7. Soyabean crop protected by homeopathic remedies. Brazil is the second largest producer of soyabean in the world after the United States with an annual production of nearly 100,000 tonnes. Over the years there has been an emergence of diseases that harms the crop and this is due to a disease known as charcoal rot. *Macrophomina phaseolina*, also known as "cotton root rot" fungus, is a pathogen that is responsible for this, but it also affects a variety of other crops, including corn, and peas besides soyabean. It can cause wilting and yellowing of plant leaves and stems, as well as root rot. The fungus can survive in soil for many months and is often resistant to conventional pesticides.

A study was conducted to evaluate the control of charcoal rot in soybean using *Sepia* and *Arsenicum album* homeopathic solutions in dynamizations of 6C, 12C, 24C, 36C and 48C. *Sepia* reduced up to 32% of the fungal growth (Lorenzetti, Stangarlin, & Kuhn, 2017).

8. Anticancer activity of homeopathic remedy *in-vitro*. One study investigated the *in-vitro* anticancer activity of homeopathic preparations of *Terminalia chebula* and evaluate their nanoparticulate nature. Mother tincture and other homeopathic preparations (3X, 6C and 30C) of *Terminalia chebula* were tested for their effect on the viability of breast cancer (MDAMB231 and MCF7) and non-cancerous (HEK 293) cell lines. Mother tincture preparation decreased the viability of breast cancer (MDAMB231 and MCF7) and non-cancerous (HEK 293) cells. However, the other potencies (3X, 6C and 30C) decreased the viability of only breast cancer cells without affecting the viability of the non-cancerous cells. All of the potencies reduced the growth kinetics of breast cancer cells, more specifically at 1:10 dilution at 24, 48 and 72 hours (Wani, Prabhune, Jadhav, Ranjekar, & Kaul-Ghanekar, 2016).

9. Inhibition of fungi associated with okra seed. Saxena and associates found that 22 genera of fungi associated with okra were inhibited when treated with *Thuja occidentalis, Acidum nitricum,* and, *Sulphur* (Saxena, Pandey, & Gupta, 1987).

How homeopathy employs the placebo

Samuel Hahnemann, the founder of homeopathy was, as far as we know, the first physician who administered placebos to his patient on a systematic and regular basis. This fact is recorded in unpublished documents, such as patients' letters in the Archives of the Institute for the History of Medicine, at the Robert Bosch Foundation in Stuttgart. His prescription rate of placebo was very high. It was between 54% and 85%, and he marked placebos with the paragraph symbol § (Jutte, 2014). Was Hahnemann trying to deceive his patients? No. These placebos were given between doses of actual remedies to allow the remedies to "unfold their action" and his patients, as was customary then, were used to a repetitive dose of medication. Homeopathy, with its underlying tenet of the minimum dose, was different, and placebo pills were used only to fill in the time gap till the next dose was due. Very often, a single dose of remedy was sufficient to affect a cure.

Inference

From the foregoing it will be seen that the strawman arguments against homeopathic action of remedies stand demolished.

CHAPTER 16

Patient, Practitioner and Remedy Entanglement

"Before operating on a patient's brain, I realized, I must first understand his mind: his identity, his values, what makes his life worth living, & what devastation makes it reasonable to let that life end.

– Paul Kalanithi

When Breath Becomes Air

Dr. Lionel Milgrom, a British chemist and former member of the teaching faculty at the Imperial College London is a practicing homeopath. He has suggested that one must understand that homeopathy rests on the triad of the intimate interactions or "entanglement" between the Patient, the Practitioner and the selected Remedy. This can be best understood with an example. A petri dish containing a living culture of Methicillin-Resistant Staphylococcus Aureus (MRSA) bacteria is not a disease until it infects a patient and is diagnosed by a practitioner. Thus, there is an intimate correlation (entanglement) between diseased patients, remedies, and practitioners.

Conventional medical science has attempted to factor out all these essentially entangled entities into clear-cut separate (and empirically testable) elements. The result of this reductionist programme is the increasing emphasis on molecular pharmacology (at the expense of the human interaction between the patient and the practitioner) as the only factor really worthy of consideration in disease processes. This is not to say that molecular pharmacology is wrong. However, by concentrating only on local interactions, e.g., the spatial-temporal interactions of small drug-molecules with cellular 'receptor sites' is an incomplete and myopic view (Milgrom, 2003).

Biomedicine has fostered a process called "medicalization" whereby medicine has become an economic commodity for the for the benefit of the profit-making medical care industry. Virtually every normal, daily human experience, be it birth and death, sadness and grief, variation in physiological parameters in response to daily challenges have been medicalised. Another source of patients' disappointment with biomedicine is its limited efficacy in cases of chronic disease and the side-effects of its drugs. It may sound harsh, but the role of the physician has been reduced to that of a technician to fix parts of the body or as a delivery agent of drugs. The element of care is sadly missing in today's practice of medicine. Patient-centeredness respects patients' wishes and allows active patient participation and is therefore related to improved outcomes.

Doctors Prefers Nurse Practitioner over an MD!

Today, the physician-patient interaction is unequal, and any social relationship based on a power imbalance is unfair. Physicians dictate the rules of this relationship through monopolisation of information, conferred status and money. The patients are expected to comply without questioning the medical "authority". Submitting to the hegemony of the physician and passively and uncritically agreeing to this power imbalance reinforces the hegemony.

Dr. Sunil Dhand, MD, is a US based British doctor and is an active influencer on the social media. He feels that the western medical model is collapsing, and he has *"completely lost faith in the medical profession."* He says that if he were in a situation where he needed to see a doctor for any ailment that he could not resolve himself, he would rather consult a Nurse Practitioner (NP) or a Physician Assistant (PA), than a doctor. He found that most of them were in fact better than the MD qualified doctors. He feels medical education teaches "a load of nonsense" and that it should be cut by half. According to him this applies even in specialist care. He found many people have had better experience with NPs and PAs, who are generally more observant, more empathetic, have a more positive outlook, and are better listeners. Naturally, his comments and posts on YouTube and Twitter (now X) were met with an outrage from some mainstream practitioners, but there was a deluge of support from not just laypersons but from medical doctors as well. Dr. Dhand goes on to speak highly of homeopathy (Dhand, 2023).

What makes homeopathy different?

We have referred to the biopsychosocial model (BSP) of medicine earlier. The homeopathic model incorporates the principles of BSP and is based on holism and comprehension of the totality of the patient. It uses patient-centred communication with a high degree of physician cooperation, empathy, hopefulness, enablement, and narrative competence, all of which can improve outcomes. For this reason, patients are increasingly attracted to homeopathy. The medical establishment finds it difficult to discern why patients still turn to homeopathy with the high degree of satisfaction consistently reported across a broad range of diseases.

It has been found that patients suffering from allergies or asthma would continue treatment only if they felt the physician was giving them enough time and attention at follow-up consultations. Optimism was also described by participants in some studies as an important characteristic that emerges from consultations with homeopaths. Others also found that patients could open up and unload their hearts and explore their issues (Viksveen P. R., 2017).

Therefore, it is important to understand how homeopaths conduct their consultation and what their communication styles are. This is so because both the observed clinical effects and the positive subjective experiences reported by patients is remarkable. This is supported by findings from a recent clinical trial of homeopathy in rheumatoid arthritis (RA) patients. It confirmed that the clinical benefits arose from the consultation and not the remedy. Four themes associated with improved coping were, (i) receiving emotional support; (ii) exploring the illness; (iii) exploring self; and (iv) gaining advice. Exploring the wider narrative of their illness, enabled participants to address their individual needs and for some, this process of increased awareness changed their perception resulting in the perceived benefits (Brien, Leydon, & Lewith, 2012).

It is indeed ironical that western medicine which traces its origins to Greek medicine and philosophy has lost its connection with their roots. Aesclepius was the Greek God of Healing and Medicine. He was married to Epione (Goddess of Soothing Pain), who gave him five immortal daughters and two mortal sons. His daughters, Hygeia (Goddess of Disease Prevention), Aceso (Goddess of Recovery), Iaso (Goddess of Recovery), Aegle (Goddess of Recuperation), and Panacea (Goddess of Universal Remedy), represented the stages of the healing process and medicinal treatment. His mortal sons were Machaon and Podalirius, while the former was the father of surgery (Healer of Trauma), the latter was a physician (Healer of Unseen Evils). Epione and her immortal daughters represented the essential (immortal) stages of healing, which are applicable even today, yet have been driven into oblivion and this tradition has been painted as witchcraft and superstition.

Doctor, Heal Thyself

It has been confirmed that humanistic interactions with patients are very fulfilling experiences for patients and engender trust with the doctor. But such engagements also provide the doctor job satisfaction and prevent burnout among physicians.

Most modern Western medicine practitioners do not distinguish the difference between suffering and illness. A person experiences suffering as a whole, not in parts. It is not limited to his or her body or body part and has its source in the threat to the intactness of the person as a complex social and psychological entity. Therefore, it is the duty of the physician to provide relief for both the illness as well as suffering. A physician's failure to understand the nature of suffering can result in a medical intervention that though technically adequate, fails to relieve suffering and could become a source of suffering itself.

Today, medical pedagogy encourages "detached concern" which devalues subjectivity, emotion, relationship, and solidarity to nothingness. Empathy is the naturally occurring subjective experience of similarity between the feelings expressed by self and others without losing sight of whose feelings belong to whom. When a physician exercises detached concern, he is overlooking even a minimal recognition and understanding of the patient's emotional state. To rectify the situation "medical humanities", which encompasses ethics, social science, and arts, should be incorporated as an important component of medical education.

In contrast to the situation described above, homeopathy practitioners have an entirely different approach. During a typically long consultation practitioners of homeopathy ask patients broad questions to elicit subjective symptoms and life experiences, and this enables them to develop a deeper understanding of the "inner world" of the patient and acts as a tool to connect psychological and physiological symptoms. The remedy is then selected based on the patients individual set of symptoms. This sets the recovery process in motion by stimulating the patient's self-healing powers or Vital Force. This holistic approach gives patients an expectation that it will address the cause of their illness, and enable treatment based on their individual experiences, and also provide a non-reductionist explanatory framework for their illness.

A study conducted at the University of Westminster investigated the experiences of users of complementary and alternative medicine (CAM) using a qualitative approach. In-depth interviews were conducted with 11 frequent users and analysed using Interpretative Phenomenological Analysis (IPA). Results indicated that the patient-practitioner relationship and explanatory frameworks provided by CAM were perceived as important components of the therapeutic process, irrespective of treatment efficacy. CAM served a variety of functions beyond the explicit relief of symptoms by increasing energy and relaxation, facilitating coping, and enhancing self/other awareness. It is therefore important that these wider effects are taken into account when evaluating complementary medicine in order to reflect patients' experiences accurately (Cartwright & Torr, 2005).

Sadly, debates centred around homeopathy are focussed only on its contentious medical approach with criticism and arguments about the nature of the active ingredient of ultra-molecular doses and the mechanism for their action. This is altogether unfounded because it has been demonstrated that ultra-molecular doses exert influence in animal, plant, soil and *in-vitro*.

Many patients refer to homeopathic treatment as being part of a long-term journey of self-discovery *for both the patient and practitioner* as many patients did not know what the underlying reason for their illness was. Thus, a homeopathic consultation is a collaborative engagement. Many practitioners feel that their own life experiences contributed to being able to understand their patients – a phenomenon often described as the "wounded healer", a term created by the celebrated and renowned psychologist Carl Jung.

Dr. Arthur Kleinman, MD, found that wounded healers have an increased sensitivity to patient needs, have better communication skills, and have more genuine empathy. Moreover, many used their personal experiences (both bad and good) to change their clinical practice to reflect the kind of care they would have wanted as patients (Kleinman, 2020). Would the suffering be the same for a particular named disease if the person were an obese hypersensitive mother of six, with no family support, no job be comparable to a Beverly Hills socialite? The Greeks had two words to describe this dichotomy – *pathos* versus *ponos*, that is the suffering versus disease.

Hans Selye, one of the first to extensively study the physiological and psychological effects of stress on the human body, had noted during his student days that patient suffering from different diseases often exhibited identical signs and symptoms! That is very close to the teachings of homeopathy as propounded by Samuel Hahnemann who considered subjective, idiosyncratic symptoms to be the key to finding the most suitable remedy (Hahnemann, 2013). That is what makes homeopathy unique because it integrates patient and practitioner experience with the remedy which reflects the experiential reality of the person seeking cure.

CHAPTER 17

"Explaining" Homeopathy

"It's easier to learn things for life by the age of 12 and not the age of 18. This is just my guess."

– Luc Montagnier, Nobel Laureate

Homeopathy is controversial because medicines in high potencies such as those designated as 30C and 200C involve very high dilution factors ($1:10^{60}$ and $1:10^{400}$ respectively) which are many orders of magnitude greater than Avogadro's number, so that theoretically there should be no measurable remnants of the starting materials. To quickly recount what this means, the Avogadro's limit refers to the concentration below which a solution becomes so dilute it is unlikely that any of the original molecules are present. More precisely, we can define the limit as the concentration at which there is only one molecule per litre of solution. Since there are 6.022×10^{23} atoms in a mole, this gives a limit of 1.66×10^{-24} mol/L. From a probabilistic point of view, we could say that at concentrations well above Avogadro's limit (1.66×10^{-24} mol/L) the probability of obtaining at least one molecule tends towards unity but falls off quickly below the limit.

However, it is a historical fact that Dr. Samuel Hahnemann had discovered that through serial dilutions of medicinal substances, carried out in steps, and accompanied by vigorous shaking known as 'succussion' at each dilution step, elicited some kind of a potent activity to these solutions. This unique technique is termed by homeopaths as "potentization".

What this means is that there is need to reorient the thinking in this regard. This means shifting one's way of thinking about a deeply entrenched concept. Even today, mainstream science and scientists suffer from the same bias the Church once held against Giordano Bruno and Galileo Galilei in th 16th century. Bruno's trial reflected a tension between religion and philosophy, while Galileo's trial reflected a tension between religion and science. Today we can see parallels when it comes to arguments against homeopathy from mainstream medicine.

The Benveniste *Affair*

Dr. Jacques Benveniste (1935-2004) was a French immunologist. He qualified as a physician in 1960 and practised medicine in Paris before taking a research job in cancer at the Scripps Clinic in California. Later he returned to France and was appointed as the head of allergy and inflammation immunology at the French biomedical research agency INSERM. He is best known for his discovery of *platelet-activating factor* and its relationship with histamine and the role it plays in inflammatory response.

A member of Benveniste's staff put a homoeopathically diluted remedy through his allergy test, and it returned a positive result! Therefore, Benveniste began experimenting to confirm these findings. He published his findings in the prestigious science journal *Nature* in 1988 describing the action of very high dilutions of anti-IgE antibody on the degranulation of human basophils. These results were published in *Nature* and biologists were puzzled by Benveniste's results, because "only molecules of water, and no molecules of the original antibody remained in these high dilutions". However, Benveniste concluded that the configuration of molecules in water was biologically active, as was demonstrated by its action. Following this a journalist coined the word *memory of water* for this phenomenon. Benveniste had followed all accepted scientific practices, and he asked other laboratories to try and replicate the findings. In 1988, scientists from six laboratories in four countries (France, Canada, Israel and Italy) coauthored an article showing that highly diluted antibodies could cause basophil degranulation. This was established under stringent experimental conditions such as blind double-coded procedures. Further, the experimental dilution (anti-IgE) and the control one (anti-IgG) were prepared in exactly the same manner, with the same number of dilution and agitation sequences (Thomas, 2007).

The reaction of the mainstream was vicious and rabid. *Nature's* referees could not fault Benveniste's experimental procedures and also could not comprehend his results. Hence mainstream scientists not only attacked it as being an unrealistic hypothesis, but also challenged that a panel of three members would try and replicate the results. Surprisingly, the panel of three had only one "scientist", Sir John Maddox, a popular science writer, a sceptic Walter Stewart and a stage magician-turned-crusader James Randi! These three made seven attempts to replicate the Benveniste study, and in four of them they proved to be favourable. But the team of sceptics expressed that they were *not satisfied with the rigour of the methodology.*

We have mentioned about Dr. John Ioannidis, an epidemiologist at George Washington University earlier in this book. He conducted a study on the validity of certain research findings and found that as much as 90% of published medical information is flawed, plain wrong or nonsense. The major three types of misconduct (falsification, fabrication and plagiarism) are categorized as "scientific dishonesty". Minor breaches of "responsible conduct of research" (bad practice) include concealed double publication, dubious accreditation as author, "salami" publication etc. As a matter of fact, *Nature* itself reported that manipulation of data, which it termed "grey zone" behaviour, is common among scientists (Lose & Klarskov, 2017).

The matter did not die down but was simply kept wrapped under the sheets, until another European multi-centre study published in 1999 showed results similar to Benveniste. And, in a strategically planned move it ignored the findings of the Benveniste study, and there was not a whimper of protest this time. The strategy was to allow the matter to remain buried.

In these experiments, degranulation was provoked with substantial doses of IgE, a concentration of 0.04 moles/ml was used. Then, the test treatments were performed with potencies 15C, 16C, 17C, 18C and 19C (centesimal dilutions beyond the Avogadro's Limit) of histamine hydrochloride in distilled water, prepared with vortexing. Comparison was made with blinded controls administered with distilled water. The experiments were conducted in parallel at 4 independent laboratories. Coordination, coding, randomisation and statistical analysis were done by the Belgian group. Participants received preliminary training in the method and all reagents came from the same source. The pooled results from the 4 laboratories yielded a total of 772 valid data points (Belon, et al., 1999). The presentation of this paper was low-key, and not surprisingly, in view of the preceding controversy, and as a precaution the Benveniste's *Nature* paper was not even cited!

Certainly, the researchers deserve congratulations and kudos for persisting and venturing into such a controversial minefield years after the controversy. It also proves that fact-twisting, errors, omissions, misquotations and mistruths are symptoms of a crusade by the hegemonic structure based on the triad of the insurance, pharmaceutical and hospital industry, supported by various non-statutory medical associations worldwide.

Dr. Luc Montagnier, the Noble Nobel Laureate

Dr. Luc Montagnier (1932-2022) was a French virologist and a noble laureate who co-discovered the human immunodeficiency virus (HIV) and hepatitis B virus (HBV). He was awarded the Nobel Prize in Physiology and Medicine in 2008, for this discovery. Montagnier made significant contributions to the fields of virology and molecular biology, and his discoveries have had a significant impact on public health. He continued researching and developing new treatments for HIV throughout his career.

On 28 June 2010, Montagnier spoke at the Lindau Nobel Laureate Meeting in Germany where 60 Nobel Prize winners had gathered, along with 700 other scientists to discuss the latest breakthroughs in medicine, chemistry and physics. He stunned his audience when he presented a new method for detecting viral infections that bore close parallels to the basic tenets of homeopathy. Montagnier's comments were rapidly embraced by homeopaths eager for greater credibility.

In the interview to the prestigious *Science* magazine, he stated that Jacques Benveniste, whose controversial homeopathic work had been discredited, was "a modern Galileo". When asked if he was not "worried that your colleagues will think you have drifted into pseudo-science?", he replied: "No, because it's not pseudoscience. It's not quackery. These are real phenomena which deserve further research.

Montagnier was also questioned on his beliefs about homeopathy, to which he replied: "I can't say that homeopathy is right in everything. What I can say now is that the high dilutions are right. High dilutions of something are not nothing. They are water structures which mimic the original molecules. We find that with DNA, we cannot work at the extremely high dilutions used in homeopathy; we cannot go further than a 10^{-18} dilution, or we lose the signal. But even at 10^{-18}, you can calculate that there is not a single molecule of DNA left. And yet we detect a signal." (Science, 2010).

Ridicule in the History of Science

The history of science is filled with examples of ridicule and scepticism towards new ideas. Throughout history, scientists and innovators have been met with criticism and ridicule for their groundbreaking discoveries and theories. However, over time, these ideas have been proven true and have led to significant advancements in various fields. It is important to remember that science is a process of inquiry and experimentation, and new ideas should be evaluated based on their merits and evidence, rather than being dismissed outright. Ignaz Semmelweis was ridiculed when he proposed that in hospitals death toll could be lowered by doctors washing their hands between patients. After years of trying, he finally gave up and ended his days in an insane asylum. It wasn't until around 20 years later that Louis Pasteur's germ theory caught on and more people took to wash their hands as suggested by Semmelweis. Gregor Mendel's work that laid the foundation of the science of genetics was noticed only 16 years after his death, and 34 years after it was first published.

What was the underlying reason for rejecting such great ideas which seem so obvious today? Resistance to new ideas seems to be an enduring human characteristic, and scientists, despite extolling the virtues of objectivity have often proved themselves very "human" in this respect. One must admit that ridicule is a serious and endemic problem in science.

Nanoparticle Research – Defying the Avogadro's Bogeyman

The Indian Institutes of Technology (IIT) are a group of prestigious public technical universities in India. There are currently 23 IITs in India, located in different states of the country. These institutions are considered amongst the best technical institutions in the world. Some of the famous alumni of IITs include the industrial magnate Ratan Naval Tata, physicist Abhijit Banerjee, mathematician Madhav Gopakumar, the early internet pioneer Yogen Dalal and Google CEO Sundar Pichai. These alumni have made significant contributions to their respective fields and have held key positions in various industries and organizations across the world. The IITs are at the leading edge of technologies in various domains such as computer science, robotics, artificial intelligence (AI), data science, biotechnology, green energy, and other emerging fields.

Given the international repute they enjoy, any research coming from an IIT is taken seriously the world over.

A team of researchers found that extreme homeopathic dilutions retain the properties of the starting materials well beyond the limits imposed by the Avogadro's number. There is no hypothesis which predicts the retention of properties of starting materials at dilution factors of $1:10^{60}$ and $1:10^{400}$. So far, no physical entity been shown to exist in these high potency medicines. For the first time it has been demonstrated by Transmission Electron Microscopy (TEM), electron diffraction and chemical analysis by Inductively Coupled Plasma-Atomic Emission Spectroscopy (ICP-AES), that physical entities exist in these extreme dilutions, in the form of nanoparticles of the starting metals and their aggregates (Chikramane, Suresh, Bellare, & Kane, 2010).

This points to the fact that chemistry of substances at ultra-high dilutions is akin to the behaviour of nanoscale particles, which do not display the classical diffusive behaviour of molecules and do not comply with laws of distribution in a solvent according to Dalton's atomic principle and hence Avogadro's Law (Chirumbolo, 2011). For example, gold is known as a shiny, yellow noble metal that does not tarnish, has a face centred cubic structure, is non-magnetic and melts at 1336 K. However, a small sample of the same gold is quite different, providing it is tiny enough: a 10-nanometre particle absorbs green light and thus appear red! The melting temperature decreases dramatically as the size goes down. Moreover, gold ceases to be noble, and 2-3 nm nanoparticles are excellent catalysts which also exhibit considerable magnetism. At this size they are still metallic, but smaller ones turn into insulators (Roduner, 2006). Perhaps this explains the action of a homeopathic remedy where the simple properties of the original substance are modified and effectively target a spectrum of symptoms. This points to the fact that while active ingredients are unlikely to be present in homeopathic dilutions that surpass the Avogadro limit, responses of biological systems to these substances are possible.

Effective but unimaginable treatment: Malariotherapy

What you will now read may surprise many. Imagine a person is suffering from an "incurable" disease. The treatment protocol followed in some of the top hospitals is to *infect the patient with 10 ml of screened blood from malaria patients.* Allow 3 weeks to follow with 10 to 12 fevers. Lo and behold – the patient is cured! What remains is only a patient with malaria who is then treated with quinine. This treatment was in use between 1918 and 1975. The "infected" blood was supplied by Johns Hopkins Hospital in the US and Horton Hospital, Epsom in the United Kingdom.

What is described above is a short summary of *malariotherapy.* Briefly, Malariotherapy refers to a treatment using the malaria parasite. It involves the deliberate introduction of a weakened form of the parasite into the bloodstream, with the aim of stimulating the body's immune system to develop resistance to disease.

The proponent of this therapy was Dr. Julius Wagner-Jauregg (1857-1940) who was awarded the Nobel Prize for Medicine in 1927. The Nobel citation stated that the award was for *"his discovery of the therapeutic value of malaria inoculation in the treatment of dementia paralytica"* (The Nobel Prize Foundation, 2023). Dr. Jauregg was looking for a cure of neurosyphilis, which defied treatment. There was no gold standard available at the time for diagnosis. The tests suffered from low sensitivity and culturing the fragile organism was cumbersome. Further, antibiotics had poor penetration across the Blood-Brain Barrier. How did it work?

It was only in the 1980, after the treatment went out of fashion that it was discovered that malaria causes the immune system to increase production of immune substances, namely, interleukins and interferons. This was confirmed in studies on HIV patients in regions of the world where malaria was endemic. The US Centres for Disease Control and Protection (CDC) reported that studies in Kinshasa, Congo showed that in a sample population of children who were symptomatic, no deaths were reported in children with malaria while those who were not infected with malaria reported 33 deaths. Nebraska University and the US Navy, in three independent studies, conducted in Venezuela, Indonesia and Philippines reported that in malaria infested areas people had HIV antibodies, but no AIDS, whereas AIDS existed in all non-malarial regions.

It is to be noted that Dr. Henry Heimlich (1920-2016), who developed the famous Heimlich Manoeuvre used for rescuing persons who are choking conducted further research in this field. He was not granted permission to do any field studies in the US, but was able to conduct the study in China under the auspices of Department of AIDS Control and Prevention, Guangzhou Centre for Disease Control and Prevention, Guangzhou.

The use of malariotherapy lost its popularity after antibiotics like penicillin became available and opened the floodgates of profits for pharmaceutical corporations.

The discovery of Jauregg proved what Hahnemann had stated very clearly as the cardinal principle of cure in homeopathy. Hahnemann states in the Organon that "dissimilar diseases, that meet in an organism, would not just fuse, but would either keep away or suspend one another, or if equally strong they would exist side by side and so form a complex disease". He had observed that while cowpox prevented smallpox, it suspended scarlet fever. Smallpox suspended measles. Likewise, mania suspended tuberculosis, and ringworm suspended epilepsy. Mumps too disappeared with cowpox (Hahnemann, 2013). For his discoveries Hahnemann was made into an outcaste by the medical establishment and was hounded out of town, while Jauregg was rewarded with a Nobel Prize. The Nobel Prize of 1927 was the greatest tribute to the proof of homeopathic philosophy's explanation of cure of infectious diseases.

CHAPTER 18

Medicine for the Whole Person

"There are so many ways to heal. Arrogance may have a place in technology, but not in healing. I need to get out of my own way if I am to heal."

– Dr. Anne Wilson Schaef (1934-2020)
Clinical psychologist & author of 18 best-selling books

Limits to present-day medicine

One needs to understand why contemporary medical practice is failing us. It has no cure for acute infectious diseases like influenza, SARS, MERS, HIV/AIDS, HPV or Covid-19. Similarly, the list of diseases or chronic conditions that are declared incurable by allopathy include, and are not limited to cancer, stroke, diabetes, heart disease, dementia, including Alzheimer's disease, obesity, arthritis, multiple sclerosis, and many more.

The root cause of this is the reductionist approach to life sciences. Biology has been reduced to molecular interactions, molecular biology to simple chemistry and physics and all life processes are reduced to simple laws of thermodynamics. It fails to see life systems as complex systems. The focus has been on finding a singular factor. It considers the human body as a collection of components, lie a machine. Consequently, each disease has a potential singular target for treatment – for example, if there is gastrointestinal bleeding, look for an ulcer or cancer, then attack the tumour. Disease, and not the person affected by it, becomes the central focus – as to how do a person's sleeping habits, diet, living condition, comorbidities, and stress collectively contribute to his/her heart disease, remain largely unanswered.

Homeostasis – Roots of Adaptation

In present-times any biological approach that departs from the reductionist viewpoint mentioned above is automatically deemed to be unscientific. Thus, concepts and properties of living systems that include purposefulness, design, and intentionality are overlooked or deemed as outdated concepts rooted in an archaic concept of Vitalism. It is indeed possible to integrate the ideas of Vitalism with modern concepts through the phenomenon of homeostasis to overcome the shortcomings of allopathy. Homeostasis was introduced as biological concept by the American physiologist Professor Walter Bradford Cannon, of the Harvard Medical School in 1929 (Cannon, 1929). The newly coined term referred to those activities which tend to keep the variables of a vital system constant, or within acceptable limits. Much earlier Dr. Samuel Hahnemann had laid the foundation of homeopathy as a medical system based on this action and reaction principle.

Both Cannon, and Hahnemann before him, supported the idea that natural powers, by a *vis medicatrix naturae* (the healing power of Nature), which implied the existence of agencies ready to operate correctively when the normal state of the organism is upset.

It is often forgotten that physiology is all about homeostasis. Illness occurs when homeostasis is disrupted. All chronic, acquired diseases result when normal physiologic control goes awry. It may thus be viewed as failure of homeostasis. However, while nearly every process in human physiology relies on homeostatic mechanisms for stability, happily only few have demonstrated vulnerability to dysregulation.

It is possible that during the course of evolution our genes selected, preserved and passed on to every successive generation those genes that protected us from starvation, infections, injury, and predation, and may be now, in the absence of some of these challenges, contribute to the increasing incidence of the so-called incurable diseases mentioned above.

Homeostasis can be seen at work in our body in terms of primary and secondary actions of external stimuli. The primary action is the effect which occurs in the body due to the external agent, and the secondary action is the effect observed in terms of the body's reaction to the external agent. Hence, we can also call the function of homeostasis as the "homeodynamic" response. That is why the immediate homeodynamic reaction of the body to conventional treatments gives rise to more unrelated symptoms, and hence the disease does not cure permanently.

The healing power of Nature has traditionally been defined as an internal healing response designed to restore health. Almost a century ago, famed biologist and naturalist Sir John Arthur Thomson (1861-1933) provided an additional interpretation of the word nature within the context of *vis medicatrix naturae*, defining it instead as the "natural, non-built external environment". He maintained that the healing power of nature is also that associated with mindful contact with the animate and inanimate natural portions of the outdoor environment. It is now accepted that interacting biological systems do not evolve independently. Organisms neither evolve in isolation nor simply adapt to 'external' factors. Organisms too modify their environment according to their own needs. Thus, organisms and environment undergo a continuous process of mutual interaction. This is the observed phenomenon of co-adaptation and co-evolution. This concept was first introduced by Niels Bohr, a Danish physicist, in the 1930s and later developed into a mathematical model (Galtier & Dutheil, 2007).

A good understanding of *vis medicatrix naturae* underlies the founding principles of homeopathy because the principle of similarity of medicinal substances or the Law of Similars, mentioned earlier in this book, reflects observed phenomenon of the inversion or reversal of pharmacological effects in healthy subjects as compared with sick ones. From the clinical standpoint, the medicinal substance with similarity can be regarded as a cardinal principle. According to this principle the detailed knowledge of pathogenic effects of drugs, associated with careful analysis of signs and symptoms of the person in sickness, can assist in identifying homeopathic remedies with high grade of specificity for the individual case. This has been explained earlier in the chapter on Homeopathic Pathogenetic Trials (HPTs). Hahnemann's principles have withstood the test of time and have been supported by scientific findings in an array of fields, including that of immuno-allergology, as described earlier.

Curing versus Healing

This brings us to the main topic of this chapter. It is not about fixing the human being in parts or even restoring homeostasis based on a parameter which is a statistical mean or median value of a given population without taking into account race, ethnicity, psycho-socio-economic backgrounds and other such factors. Whole Person Healing begins by going to the level of the spirit first, the mind next and then the body and organs. This is so because, in the natural world there is no mind-body-spirit split – everything is part of the whole. The split that is apparent is rooted in the history of science and the split between the Church and Science.

As a matter of fact, the so-called Evidence Based Medicine or EBM is not at all scientific! It would fail the test of acceptance as evidence in a criminal court because studies are done on heterogeneous groups of people, but the results of the studies are then applied to patients who are not representative of those groups. Thus, the currently rigid and narrow views being expressed by mainstream science are far from perfect.

Healing, on the contrary, is quite distinct from curing. Healing is the desired goal anytime a person goes to a doctor. Curing is a limited action focussed on eradicating a disease or to correct a problem. Thus, curing has a clearcut objective. The outcome can be assessed or measured. Healing is linked to restoring a sense of wholeness and wellness, which should be the aim of every healthcare practitioner. Healing is a complex process, while curing may at best be complicated. In a complicated process we have a detailed plan to follow with a step-by-step procedure to achieve the desired outcome. In a complex process there is no predictable blueprint, and the process may involve numerous variables. An example of a complicated process is sending a spacecraft to the moon, whereas a complex process can be likened to raising a child!

Therefore, an interdisciplinary healing approach to relieve pain and suffering must be evolved. Such an approach will incorporate various disciples like Homeopathy, Ayurveda, nutrition, and numerous others complimentary therapies. It is encouraging to note that this need has been recognised and increasingly several master's degree programmes are now available in the West, particularly in the US to prepare psychiatric nurses in the blended role of clinical specialist (CS) and nurse practitioner (NP). Such courses provide education to integrate mind-body interactions in therapeutic practice (Edmands, Hoff, Kaylor, Mower, & Sorrell, 2013).

To illustrate the difference between curing and healing, we can take a few examples of the objectives each address.

From the patient's point of view, the cure is sought for relief from symptoms or some dysfunction. Whereas healing provides for relief from suffering. From the physician's point of view, the focus is on the disease, while the healing happens to the person with the illness. The communication that happens in a clinical setup is largely content driven, digital and conscious. Whereas in an environment oriented for healing the communication is based on developing a relationship, the information is narrative based and at a sub-conscious level. The skills of a clinician are scientific and prescriptive, whereas a healer's approach is artistic.

It is unfortunate that modern medicine has vacated the space of the Healer to complementary and alternative therapy practitioners.

CHAPTER 19

Narrative-Based Medicine – Homeopathy Showed the Path

"Medicine, I said, begins with storytelling. Patients tell stories to describe illness; doctors tell stories to understand it. Science tells its own story to explain diseases."

– Dr. Siddharth Mukherjee, physician,
biologist and author

Modern narrative-based medicine (NBM) is a patient-centred approach to healthcare that uses storytelling and narrative technique to improve the communication and understanding of patients' medical experiences. It emphasizes the importance of listening to patients' stories and treating them as active participants in their own healthcare. The goal of narrative-based medicine is to foster empathy, build rapport, and improve the quality of care by promoting an understanding of the patient's perspective and experiences. It is a relatively new and emerging field, with research and clinical practices continuing to evolve.

NBM evolved from the confluence of ideas from apparently disparate schools of thought. It included medical humanities (history, philosophy, ethics, literature, literary theory, the arts, and cultural studies), primary care and patient-centred care, biopsychosocial medicine and holistic care, and psychoanalysis and the work of Michael Balint (Charon, 2008). The name narrative-based was deliberately selected to distinguish it from evidence-based medicine (EBM), was propagated to counteract the shortcomings of EBM. EBM is essentially the doctor's narrative of the patient's illness. By contrast, narratives incorporate the question of causality and thus foster an understanding of the patient's illness perception – something that is missing in EBM. But can narratives be considered at par with the gold standards of EBM?

According to Viktor von Weizsäcker, the illness narrative is not only a description of something pathological - it is the description of the "life of the illness" in that specific individual human being (Konnitzer, 2005). Michael Balint (1903-1978) was a Hungarian born British physician, who is known for his influential work on narrative and the doctor-patient relationship, which focused on the importance of language, storytelling, and shared narratives in the healing process. Balint's approach emphasized the importance of understanding and communicating the patient's story in order to provide better care and build a stronger therapeutic relationship. This work was furthered by Rita Charon and John Launer.

Narrative-based medicine, shifts the focus to the patient narrative, and fundamentally changes the doctor's stance toward the patient so that the doctor's focus becomes "attentive listening" and "the need to understand," rather than "the need to problem solve." However, there is no accepted definition of NBM (Solomon, 2015).

Homeopathy is Narrative Medicine

The ideas of narrative-based medicine in Western medicine are less than a century old but have been an integral part of homeopathic case-taking from the beginning. It should be borne in mind that homeopathic prescription is not subject to the same biochemical pathways as pharmacological medication and the portrait of the patient can only be complete after creating a collage from the patient's narrative of not just disease symptoms, but like and dislikes, aversions and cravings, and the story of the patient's journey of illness.

Increasingly, more people are writing autobiographical accounts of their experience of illness. This genre of writing is called "autopathography" or simply, pathography and is immensely popular because they articulate the hopes, fears and anxieties so common to sickness while providing the reader with an idea of what to expect in the journey of illness and treatment. Since pathographies are so popular, doctors read them too just to see what makes them so compelling to their patients. What is overlooked is the fact that the medical system has depersonalised sickness and writing these accounts create the space for the storytelling or narrative the patients wish to express. In fact, the pathography can be seen as complementing a patient's medical record (Hunter, 1991). The common denominator of all pathographies, whatever the ostensible motives of their authors, is that the act of writing in some way seems to facilitate recovery: the healing of the whole person (Hunsaker, 1999).

Homeopathy, like narrative medicine, is a medical approach that emphasizes the use of storytelling and patient experiences in understanding and treating health issues. The key to homeopathic approach is using and understanding metaphors used in the language of the patient. This is classified as "analogue communication" because in metaphorical language the metaphor expresses a similarity between what is expressed, and the expression used. Complex concepts relating to illness and health can be expressed by metaphors. Neurolinguists point out that metaphors have both a bodily and a cultural root. Metaphors help to understand an "illness narrative".

It is now increasingly felt that physical symptoms are often a manifestation of emotional or mental imbalances, and that healing the underlying emotional and mental issues can lead to lasting physical health.

Homeopathy offers that unique opportunity without resorting to psychotropic drugs. That is possible because, as we have seen earlier, remedies are chosen based on symptoms that they create in healthy subjects during homeopathic pathological trials (a.k.a. *provings*). It was Hahnemann who originated the concept of homeopathic healing through similarity (Hahnemann, 2013). The experience of "similarity" is bound to a specific affective mood, an interactive situation, and a remedy portrait. The 'drug picture' can be visualised as the remedy's story and the history as the patient's story metaphorizes the narrative quality of homeopathy (Konitzer, Renee, & Doering, 2003).

The Repertory

Reference has been made to homeopathic pathogenetic trials (HPTs) or *provings* in an earlier chapter. A proving is the testing of a potentized substance to find out which symptoms that substance is capable of producing, and hence curing. Provings are the pillars upon which homeopathic practice stands. Without accurate provings all prescribing indications are bound to be vague guesses at best, and pure fiction at worst. There is no other way to predict the effect of any given substance as a remedy with any degree of accuracy, and the use of signatures, toxicology or fancy ideas cannot approximate the precise knowledge gained by a thorough proving.

Once the data of *provings* is collated, it is organised in an anatomical order. This data is recorded in what is known as the Pure Materia Medica. From the Pure Materia Medica are built more readable and concise materia medicas. It takes meticulous labour over the course of many years (or generations of homeopaths) to create these materia medicas, which also include clinical symptoms in addition to the *proving* symptoms. These materia medicas are comprehensive reference books that list all of the symptoms and diseases for homeopathic remedies.

However, any detailed materia medica is an unwieldy tool. There are many remedies that share the same symptoms. For example, *Arsenicum* album has over 3,000 pathogenetic symptoms, and Sulphur has 4,000, and they share many hundreds of common symptoms. In clinical practice, physicians deal with patient symptoms, so, they would rather have a handy tool that allows them to quicky access all the remedies that exhibit the symptom that is of interest to the physician. The tool that is created by homeopaths for this purpose is known as the Repertory. Just as there are many materia medicas, there a numerous repertories. The repertory may be likened to an inventory of symptom descriptions – it may be likened to a telephone directory – it aids in searching symptoms and all the corresponding remedies. Usually, repertories list remedies in alphabetic order in different anatomical regions from head to toe. There is a large section on mind symptoms too. Naturally, to manage the volume, repertories usually summarise the symptoms, and often the proving data is not accurately reflected in a repertory.

Dr. José Mirilli and the Thematic Repertory

José Antonio Mirilli, a Brazilian homeopath and researcher organised a repertory exclusively for the symptoms of the mind. He found that most repertories organize mental symptoms in an alphabetical order, and that is not very helpful. He says, *"We could compare the mental symptoms with the bones of the human body. We can outline all the bones of a body according to the alphabetical order of their related names. Such a line of bones would be an unrecognizable organization of the human body as a whole."* Mirilli picked out principal themes of mind symptoms from the proving records (not repertories) and created a new *Thematic Repertory*. There are 300 great themes and 1,400 short word themes.

Mirilli's Thematic Repertory provides meaning to the metaphors used by the patient in narrative medicine. Afterall, of what use would a narrative be if the doctor could not find a suitable remedy for the condition? For example, if a patient becomes sick every time he is reproached, reprimanded, the corresponding Mirilli's theme would be *Censured*. Such key themes are easy to pick from the Thematic Repertory. Once the key themes are picked out, it is easy to identify the portrait of a remedy when combined with pathological symptoms, strange and peculiar symptoms,

symptoms showing a common generality (e.g., better in sunlight, worse cold drafts of air, etc.).

Let us see how the Thematic Repertory can help by examining one case-study from Dr. Mirilli's clinic. A child presented a pattern of chronic allergy, in which the main local symptom was a night cough that condemned him (and his family) to insomnia. At the evaluation of mental symptoms, the most characteristic, was that in games, he always wanted to win, and when frustrated, he suffered in excess, and because of this, he had a peculiar behaviour. In the Repertory he could not find the symptoms of a "Desire to win". Therefore, he looked for its opposite, *"to lose"*, and found it. The remedy that fits the picture is *Nux Vomica* in which the patient spent all night suffering in the process in which he could gain or lose a lot of money. Afterwards, he verified that many symptoms of *Nux Vomica* are related to ambition themes. At a later consultation he evaluated general and local symptoms. To his surprise, the best indicated remedy was *Nux Vomica* again (Mirilli, 2009).

With an understanding of Mirilli's Themes we can get a better understanding of Bach Flower Remedies discussed earlier.

CHAPTER 20

Care for the Elderly

"Caregiving can never be one-size-fits-all."

– Nancy L. Kriseman
The Mindful Caregiver

Ageing

The Italian philosopher and poet of the early Romantic period Giacomo Leopardi (1798-1837) had once remarked, *"Old age is supreme evil... We all fear death, and yet we all desire old age"*. Ageing is an inevitable part of life. After all, our cells aren't made to last forever! But why does this happen? For decades, scientists have been studying the subject. Answering the question as to why we age is equivalent to answering the question of "what is life?" itself. There are currently more than three hundred theories on why we age, and experts are learning more every day (da Costa, et al., 2016).

Most of us view ageing as a gradual, linear process. However, research suggests that the biological aging process isn't steady and appears to accelerate periodically — with the greatest bursts coming, on average, around ages 34, 60, and 78 (Collins, 2019). Aging is also associated with several chronic diseases that limit life-span.

Ageing is a complex process that varies from person to person due to genetic, lifestyle, and environmental factors. Aging also affects the way the body metabolizes and responds to medication, leading to decreased efficacy or increased side effects. In addition, poly-medicated patients have a limited knowledge of prescribed medication. People with five to six prescriptions were more likely to forget which medicines they are taking (Pérez-Jover, et al., 2018).

A typical example of medical care in the West for the ageing is poignantly summed up in the following account:

"When I accompanied my 85-year-old father to a doctor's appointment not long ago, his primary care physician (PCP) brushed off his complaints about chronic back pain, as well as my observations about his failing memory and balance problems. 'It's normal at his age', he told me. When asked about the 14 different medications and supplements he's on, the PCP quickly scanned several pages in the electronic record but decided not to make any changes since other specialists prescribed them for good reason. He mentioned that he wasn't comfortable overruling another physician, though he also wouldn't take any action on his own, like supplying him with a walker.

"My dad, sadly, is not the only elderly patient to take so many medications — and to have his doctor dismiss his concerns about them with a shrug. The problems start early in the drug treatment process: Frequently excluded from clinical trials are the very older adults the medications are meant to help — and whose changing physiology causes them to metabolize drugs differently. Similarly, some doctors fail to recognize when standard medication doses are only appropriate for much younger patients.

"One in three seniors who take five or more medications will have at least one bad drug reaction each year; two-thirds will require medical attention. And those over 65 are 2.5 times more likely to visit an emergency room for an adverse drug reaction than younger individuals."
(Seegert, 2019)

It is sad that even government health agencies like the CDC frequently lump everyone over 65 into one homogenous group. One root cause is the lack of medical training to attend to the special demands of older patients. Medical schools routinely offer rotations in specialties like paediatrics, cardiology, surgery and emergency medicine. But geriatrics? Often not on the list! Medical students do not want to specialize in elder care, which is frequently considered a "poor stepchild" to other specialties. Isn't this ironical? Most people alive today will spend more years in elderhood than in childhood, and many will be elders for 40 years or more (Aronson, 2019).

That is why during the twilight years, homeopathy can be the most suited form of care because it can be individualised. It starts by identifying the specific symptoms and ailments that a person experiences, and then provides remedies that address them. The body's ability to heal naturally through homeopathy can help to alleviate many common issues associated with aging such as pain, insomnia, and digestive problems. Homeopathic treatment is non-invasive, non-toxic, and may also be beneficial for conditions like arthritis, asthma, and heart disease in older adults. For these reasons, many elderly persons choose to receive homeopathic treatment.

Principal concerns

The principal concerns that elderly people face are, (1) absentmindedness and memory issues, (2) vision problems, (3) hearing problems and tinnitus, (4) sleeplessness, (5) coping with terminal disease, (6) recovery from surgery and dealing with bedsores that may follow, (7) constipation, (8) incontinence, (9) vertigo and loss of balance, (10) breathing problems, (11) loneliness, worry, and, (12) dealing with grief and the loss of a loved one. Besides this, the elderly may have several comorbidities, diabetes, hypertension, obesity, anxiety and other. This population is also subject to polypharmacy, with the attendant risks of unknown drug interactions.

It has been found that up to 30 per cent of hospital admissions of people aged 65 years and over are medication-related, and approximately half of these could be prevented (Roughead & Semple, 2009).

In other words, the portrait of the wholeness of a person's being is made up of numerous pixels can makes sense only when viewed holistically. This fact is ignored and the elderly are viewed through the tunnel vision of a super-specialisation oriented medical system. Homeopathy is a system that views the whole person and not merely a collection of body parts.

Homeopathy for elder patients

A study was undertaken by the internationally renowned Charité University Medical Centre, home to many Nobel Prize awardees, to find out the range of diagnoses, course of treatment and long-term outcome in elderly patients who choose to receive homeopathic medical treatment. It investigated homeopathic practice in an industrialised country under everyday conditions. The aim of the study was to determine the spectrum of diagnoses and treatments, as well as to describe the course of illness over time among older patients who chose to receive homeopathic treatment (Teut, Lüdtke, Schnabel, Willich, & Witt, 2010). This study covered 3,981 patients with a mean age of 73 years for men and 74 years for women. This prospective study also covered a follow-up over a two-year period. 98.6% of the sample population had chronic complaints like hypertension, sleep disturbance, diabetes mellitus, sciatica, low back pain, osteoarthritis and depression for over 11 years.

It was observed that patient and physician assessments of the severity of the complaints consistently demonstrated substantial improvements following homeopathic treatment, which were maintained through follow-up at 3 months, 12 months and 24 months. Overall, the quality-of-life improvement and the number of medicines taken remained stable within the 24 months observation period. The physician's assessment of severity of complaints decreased from 6.6 to 3.7 on a numerical rating scale.

The treatment was individualised, and each patient received on average 6±5 (not necessarily different) homeopathic remedies. Prescriptions were given consecutively following the principles of classical homeopathy. More than half of all prescriptions were covered by 9 homeopathic remedies. The strongest clinical improvements of complaints were described by patients in the first three months.

This only proved the efficacy of homeopathy helping the elderly patients with longstanding chronic diseases.

Another international multicentre, prospective, observational study in a real-world medical setting compared the effectiveness of homeopathy with conventional medicine. The response to treatment as measured by

1. The primary outcomes criterion for patients receiving homeopathy was as high as 82.6%, while for conventional medicine it was only 68%.
2. Improvement in less than 1 day and in 1 to 3 days was noted in 67.3% of the group receiving homeopathy and in only 56.6% of those receiving conventional medicine.
3. The adverse events for those treated with conventional medicine was as high as 22.3% versus only 7.8% for those treated with homeopathy.
4. Seventy-nine percent (nearly four out of five) of patients treated with homeopathy were very satisfied while only 65.1% (fewer than two out of three) of patients treated with conventional medicine were very satisfied.

It can be seen from the above figures that homeopathy proved to be better than conventional therapy and emphasises the necessity of integrating it with Western medicine for the sake of patients' welfare and wellbeing.

CHAPTER 21

Ars Moriendi: The Art of Dying

"The art of living well and the art of dying well are one."

– Epicurus

The *"Art of Dying"* is a concept that focuses on enhancing the quality of life in individuals who are facing the end of their life. It emphasizes the importance of palliative care and advance care planning in helping patients and their families make informed decisions about medical treatments and end-of-life care. For many, pain is often a constant companion in their journey towards death. Ultimately all of us will die, sooner or later, despite excellent care and the magnificent advances of modern medicine. Still, death is viewed as a failure of medicine rather than a certainty of Nature. Therefore, it is an opportunity to help the patients and their families to experience what has come to be called "a good death." This is in spite of the fact that death happens all the time, yet medical practice never "sees" it. Death is normal, and not something to be resisted, postponed, or avoided.

How would doctors like to die? Dr. Ken Murray, MD had conducted a survey and found that doctors do not want *"everything possible done,"* - something they often impose on their patients. Doctors don't wish to be resuscitated when death is eminent; they want to die at home immersed in the love and presence of family. Dr. Murray does believe that too much futile, expensive, and often painful end-of-life care is still practiced while a peaceful death at home or in hospice care is underused. Murray says that there is need for better protocols for hospitals and emergency medical services that often use mandatory resuscitation protocols even in the most futile and inappropriate instances (Hagan, 2015).

It is now acknowledged that "medical futility", i.e., a treatment that has less than 1% chance of success at the end of life, is a growing challenge to medicine. Medical futility was identified in the majority of case consultations. Many doctors were interviewed, and they found it futile to offer interventions that carry disproportionate risks, harms and costs (Jox, Schaider, Marckmann, & Borasio, 2012). Then why do doctors provide treatments? One of the reasons was that the treating doctors were inexperienced in handling death and dying. They had concerns about legal risk and had poor communication skills (Willmott, et al., 2016). The incidence of these treatments is not insignificant. It was around 12% (range between 6% to 19.6%) or one out of every eight of all end-of-life treatments (Carter, Winch, & Barnett, 2017).

As recently as 1945, most deaths occurred at home, but by 1980 only 17% died at home. Even those who somehow did die at home likely died too suddenly to make it to the hospital due to a massive heart attack, stroke, or violent injury, or were too isolated to get somewhere that could provide help. In the United Kingdom almost a quarter of occupied hospital bed-days are taken up by patients who are in the last year of life and some 60% of all deaths occur there. Thirty seven per cent of patients admitted to UK intensive care units die within six months. In the modern epidemic of multiple organ failure, it costs twice as much to die in an intensive care unit as it does to survive (Bion & Strunin, 1996). Indeed, the third highest cause of death in the United States is medical error. That does not mean that most of medical errors are due to inherently bad doctors. Rather, most errors represent systemic problems, including poorly coordinated care, fragmented insurance networks, the absence or underuse of safety nets, and other protocols, in addition to unwarranted variation in physician practice patterns that lack accountability (Johns Hopkins Medicine, 2016).

How can we approach death with dignity? Homeopathy can help by combining Narrative Based medicine and remedies – because dying is such an individualised and personal experience that the doctor must come out of the strait-jacket of "one size fits all" approach.

What they don't teach in Med School

Death is a topic that finds little or no mention in medical school curricula. For example, if we were to search for the word "death" in a typical MBBS syllabus, which runs into 229 pages (50,000 words or more), one could get only 35 hits, and that too the word is in the context of medico-legal aspects, issuance of death certificates, or estimating the time of death in a post-mortem examination. Out of 3950 teaching hours, only 40 hours (approximately 1%) are devoted to medical ethics, and out of 10 topics there is just one section on death and too is devoted to prolongation of life, life support, suicide and the like. Thus, all concepts of death of most medical professionals are entirely based on their faith.

Approaching Death with Homeopathy

Homeopathy's highest goal is to cure in a gentle way without causing harm (Hahnemann, 2013). Like other doctors, homeopaths too strive to save lives. However, even the best of homeopaths may not always save a life. When a patient is involved in a trauma that is life-threatening, we always give remedies based on the trauma. If it is not the person's time to leave, then all attempts to save their life will be utilized by the Vital Force.

It's not always clear when the exact moment of death occurs. A doctor or other healthcare professional will confirm the death if breathing, the heart and circulation have stopped. They may also check the eyes and body for other signs. When a person dies, those around them may notice that their face suddenly relaxes and looks peaceful. It can sometimes appear that people choose the moment to die. For example, people talk about someone hanging on until a relative arrives at their bedside. It's impossible to know why people die at the precise moment they do. However, the "pre-active" stage of dying can last around two to three weeks, but the dying process often comes into view about one to three months before death.

Some of the signs you will see in persons who are approaching death could include the following:

1. A surge of energy in the last hours of life (also known as pre-mortem surge): This can surprise family members. At this stage, your loved one may have a sudden surge of energy. They may want to get out of bed, talk to loved ones, or eat after having no appetite for days or weeks, and enhanced mental clarity that can occur hours to days before death, varying in intensity and duration (Wholihan, 2016).

2. Shallow or irregular breathing: As the moment of death comes nearer, breathing usually slows down and becomes irregular. It might stop and then start again or there might be long pauses or stops between breaths. This is known as Cheyne-Stokes breathing. This can last for a short time or long time before breathing finally stops.

3. Noisy breathing: Breathing may become loud and noisy if mucous has built up in the airways. This is because the person isn't coughing or clearing their airways. Some people call this type of breathing the death rattle because it can happen in the last days or last few hours of life.

4. Changes in appearance: One's hands and feet may start looking blotchy, purplish, or mottled. The changes in skin appearance may slowly move up their arms and legs. Also, their lips and nail beds may turn bluish or purple, and their lips may droop.

5. Unresponsiveness: At this end-of-life stage, a dying person usually becomes unresponsive. They may have their eyes open but not be able to see their surroundings. It's widely believed that hearing is the last sense to stop working. Knowing this can remind you that it's still valuable to sit with and talk to your dying loved one during this time (Blundon, Gallagher, & Ward, 2020).

6. Loss of appetite: As the body slows down to prepare for death, the metabolism slows down and requires less food. The digestive tract is also less active, which means a dying person won't feel hungry or thirsty. When a person near the end of life stops eating entirely, it is a sign that death is near. It can be as quick as a few days or up to 10 days. However, some people survive for a few weeks after they stop eating (Morrow, 2023).

Let us examine some homeopathic remedies that are useful in end-of-life care (Elements of Health, 2023).

1. *Aconite*: The person we will see intense fear, presentiment of their death, really "freaking out" with the fear. They may be very loquacious, and also have anxiety centred around the heart region.

2. *Antimonium tartaricum*: The patient may suffer high anxiety with oppression of the chest, violent pains and heaviness in the chest as if under a heavy load. They may experience suffocative anxiety and rattling of the phlegm, as if they are drowning. The sound of breathing is the characteristic "death rattle".

3. *Arsenicum album*: Well indicated for those who have difficulty letting go at the end of their lives. It probably is the remedy many homeopaths think of for the end when the patient is anxious, restless and has great fear of being alone and of course of the end. They worry about their family hey will leave behind, the distribution of their possessions and whether the house is tidy,

and when alone will dwell on their disease. They may become suspicious, obsessive and ritualistic. They are worse between midnight and 2 am. James Tyler Kent called *Arsenicum* a "friend of the dying" (Kent, 2011). He said it "gives quiet and ease to the last moments of life when given in high potency". We often talk about giving Arsenicum in high potency to help our loved ones let go of this mortal plane and cross the rainbow bridge, but a 30C may do just as well if they are ready to go and they just need a homeopathic hand to hold.

4. *Aurum metallicum*: The mental picture is of great fearfulness and anguish increasing to self-destruction, so the potential is there for suicide (or more likely talking of suicide) due to pain, etc. They are restless and need to move and can feel much worse for inactivity. They may have a delusion that they have neglected something and deserve to be punished or reproached (this is a useful remedy for PTSD in combat veterans). They can experience a great sense of responsibility, guilt and become very focused on religion at the end. They may talk about and feel better for the thought of death and they can feel much, much better for music generally.

5. *Carbo vegetabilis* is known in homeopathy as 'the corpse reviver' because in those extreme cases it either brings the patient back or allows them to pass easily. These cases are often debilitated and collapsed with weakness due to pathology in the lungs, heart, liver, congestive heart failure, etc. Generally, they are likely to have breathlessness, frequently with blue lips or face, and need a flow of air with windows open and fan on, plus they are better for sitting upright. Abdomen may be distended with flatus; cold sweat covers them, and the breath is cold.

Bringing them back is sometimes just a brief reprieve, but it can give families the opportunity to say their farewells. The great homeopath, James Tyler Kent, said to give "*Carbo veg* in water every hour for six hours, and stop, it will give rest and beatitude with many thanks." (Kent, 2011).

6. *Belladonna* is another one of our remedies for imminent death. In its plant form it is a poisonous substance which can induce vivid dreams of flying and dancing or seeing bugs or spiders climbing up the wall. It can cause mania and violence or on the other side stupor and lethargy. So, this is the picture we may see in someone who is approaching their time and in homeopathic form (where it is non-toxic!) it can help ease these sorts of symptoms.

   On the physical level, where *Belladonna* is indicated, symptoms are usually sudden. The face may be flushed with high fever, dilated pupils, along with heat, burning and redness. The heart rate and circulation are up and down, muscles weaken to a state of paralysis, blood vessels relax and the blood pressure falls leading to asphyxia and finally death. There may be desire for lemons and lemonade – and you do see this come up sometimes with Belladonna during acute illness. The patient may be very sensitive to light, noise, shiny objects and may need to lie in a dark room. They can be sensitive to drafts, especially to the head.

7. *Bryonia alba* is a useful remedy for pain. The patient is likely to be irritable, even angry due to the pain and not want to be touched. Pains are aggravated by motion and contact, with over-sensitiveness to all external impressions. Pains are likely to be pricking, darting and stinging in the joints, muscles, lungs, liver, and pain in the bones may feel as if the flesh has been beaten off.

8. *Chamomilla*, which we may think of only for teething, is a great remedy for pain. The patient may be oversensitive to the pain, which seems unendurable, driving them to despair. They are unlikely to be calm patients, but over-the-top with their reaction

to the pain, to the point of being driven crazy. As we sometimes see in labour, they can shout and curse and demand relief from their pain or their state.

9. *Lac Humanum* or mother's milk is another lovely and useful remedy at this time in a life, where it helps to make the transition beyond the veil with courage and in peace. Where souls have lost their link with God, source, spirit, etc it can help re-establish it at this time, to reduce fear. The remedy is both a link-breaker and a link-maker, so it helps in breaking the ties in order to pass over, but also bringing people together in those last stages of life if necessary.

10. *Lycopodium* is one of our classic homeopathic remedies and many will be familiar with it. I'm going to share this content as written by Mark Lambrick, the founder of Homeopathy and Palliative Care.

    "The picture is one of sudden descent into mental torture with hyperventilation. They awaken angry, sensitive and fearful. They can scream and have very ugly behaviour. Afraid to be left alone but become objectionable, domineering wanting to leave their beds but have no strength to get up. The early evenings are their worst time. Their memories weaken and they make mistakes using wrong words and confusing who they are with for people absent. They are frequently hungry, wake hungry at night, but can only eat small amounts before feeling full and have noisy flatulence. They suffer from dryness and rawness of the skin. Pale skin which is tight across the face. One foot hot and the other cold".

11. *Latrodectus mactans* is a small remedy which may be useful and one which a homeopath would likely prescribe. The remedy portrait may be seen in very anxious patients who scream with pain typically in heart failure. Cardiac pains can be violent, sharp and extend into the shoulders and both arms,

they may gasp with fear of asphyxiation and the skin may be cold as marble, all classic symptoms of angina and myocardial infarction.

12. *Lachesis* is an interesting remedy for end of life. Some of the keynote symptoms are that the patient becomes very suspicious, rambling and even malicious. They may think preparations are being made for their funeral. Not only that they may think they are already dead! They can be afraid of being poisoned, have dread of death, fear of going to bed and can be weary of life, looking at the dark side of everything. Whatever the presenting picture, at the end you would usually find that they cannot bear the clothing around their neck, chest or abdomen and you may see choking.

13. *Nitric acid*: These patients have much fear around death, great pessimism and may be weepy with discontent about self and life. They can be quarrelsome and unmoved by apologies, so unlikely to have big death-bed reconciliations as they are inclined to hold a grudge. Affinity for conditions of the mouth and anus. Blood loss, liver problems, as well as prostate and salivary issues are common and affect the appetite. Jaundice and aching in the liver may be present. There may be nausea with belching, bitter and sour vomiting, and they cannot eat anything. Better for motion but worse for the slightest touch, worse for lack of sleep, as well as cold air and hot weather.

14. *Opium* is a homeopathic remedy which is restricted for use in Australia, but I give the symptoms here as it's a picture you do see frequently at the end of life and in chronic health issues in older patients. The patient is as if in a heavy stuporous sleep or may be unconscious. They will appear sleepy even when awake and they often feel no pain, which is what homeopaths call a "keynote" symptom. Looking in one of our old but great materia medica of symptom pictures, William Boericke, another of our

great masters tells us, *"He is unable to understand or appreciate his sufferings. Frightful fancies. Thinks he is not at home. Delirious talking, with wide open eyes"*. The breathing may be noisy and irregular, with hot and damp skin. They are worse from warm applications and worse during and after sleep. It's a very useful remedy for faecal impaction, often a side-effect of opiates, and for constipation with no urge at all.

15. *Rhus tox* patients may appear confused, forgetful and thoughts are cloudy. They are anxious and fearful, suspicious of family members and fear something unspecific and terrible is going to happen. They may fear they are going to be hurt, poisoned or bumped off and all of this is worse at night, driving them to attempt to get out of bed in their agitation. All this worry and anxiety comes with great restlessness and agitation (restless legs are prominent in Rhus Tox) and they constantly move about in the bed trying to find a comfortable position. They feel cold, but may actually feel hot to the touch, and want to be kept warm. They are better sitting up in the bed and may request or feel better for a very hot bath or a hot pack. They may experience diarrhoea or urinary incontinence, so can't keep anything in. Rhus Tox is a remedy for joint and skin conditions, hence they may be very itchy with achy joints, burning eyes and a constant annoying cough. As always with Rhus Tox, symptoms are worse for rest, better for first motion and may be worse for continued motion/over exertion.

16. *Tarentula cubensis:* James Tyler Kent had said that it "soothes the dying sufferer as I have never seen any other remedy do. I have seen *Arsenic, Carbo veg, Lycopodium, Lachesis,* act kindly and quiet the last horrors, but *Tarentula cubensis* goes beyond these. The pain, the rattling in the chest, with no power to throw the mucous out; the patient has but a few hours to suffer, but he can be made quiet as with the terrible morphine

in a very few minutes by *Tarentula cubensis* in the thirtieth potency (30c)."

17. *Stramonium* presents a picture of manic delirium, praying and pleading as hallucinations distress and disturb them. This may be due to medications such as opioids, due to the organs shutting down, or it may also be due to spiritually held beliefs around what happens after death. These patients may be afraid of the dark, need company and just want to escape their terror. They may be confused and mistake people around them. Talking can be an effort and their face may distort with grimaces and muscle spasms. Muscles may twitch uncontrollably, especially of the upper body and they may suffer convulsions, through which they remain conscious. Typically they may experience very dry throat with great thirst but with a dread of water. Strangely it would seem with any complaints they suffer no pain.

    As you can imagine, for the family, this would also be a terrifying picture and not a happy way to remember a dear loved one, so remedies for shock and fright such as Aconite might be required for the family members.

18. *Sandalwood* is a lesser-known remedy which can be very useful at the end of life, taking away the fear of death and bringing the knowledge that there is no death, only life eternal. We know that its smell enhances spiritual awareness and the awareness of elementals and angelic forces, and the homeopathic remedy will bring similar connection. It's a pathfinder which will shine a light forward as well as backward, something which we know happens at the end of life as the patient reflects. It allows us to surrender and to find the point of stillness within.

    It must be emphasised that the descriptions given above are only short synoptic pictures of the remedies to illustrate the choice of remedies available in the armamentarium of the homeopath. The prescription of any remedy requires keen observation of the patient's condition, thorough knowledge of Materia Medica, experience in the art of prescribing, and importantly, compassion.

Epilogue

It is a lesson in humility to know that physicians will never have perfect or complete understanding of a patient's disease or find that elusive ultimate cure. But then, that is why the wise say - medicine is both an Art as well as a Science. What we do as clinicians and clinical investigators is based on an incomplete knowledge of disease, pathophysiology, and therapeutics. Often, our understanding of these entities, and the ways in which we define them, are no more precise than the shadows cast on a wall. Leonardo da Vinci described how artists could use light and shade to evince perceptions of three-dimensional relief in paintings. Doctors too try to do the same. In other words, our knowledge is a mere collage of perceptions. This reminds one of the famous allegorical tale of Plato's Cave which expresses the uncertainty embedded in humans' perception of the world and the objects it contains. Shadows are related to two distinct surfaces - the surface of the casting object and the surface on which the shadow is cast (Alpert, 2006).

Plato's Allegory of the Cave is a dialogue between two philosophers, Glaucon and Socrates. It shows how humans can free themselves from intellectual darkness through enlightenment and the bravery to experiment with new ideas. The cave described by Plato is underground, and humans dwell there from childhood, with fetters around their necks and legs. They cannot move their heads, nor move around, but can only see the wall of the cave in front of them. Their keepers burn a fire behind them that creates light to project images of objects on the wall. That is the only impression the dwellers get about the outside world. One day, one prisoner manages to escape and walks out of the cave and discovers a whole new world. The freed prisoner is initially angry and upset because his eyes burn in the overwhelmingly bright sunlight. But eventually, his eyes adjust, and he sees the world for what it is – it is the dawn of a beautiful new reality.

Homeopathy has been around for nearly 250 years and yet it has found resistance from current mainstream medical practice. It is time modern western medicine steps out of its Plato's Cave and frees itself from intellectual darkness of ignorance and develops the courage to experiment, adapt and utilise these ideas.

If the reader can see the light outside the cave, the purpose of this book would have been served.

References

Ahmed, N. (2005, October 31). 23 years of the discovery of Helicobacter pylori: is the debate over? *Annals of Clinical Microbiology and Antimicrobials, 4*(17). doi:10.1186/1476-0711-4-17

AIIMS. (2005). *Syllabus MBBS at the AIIMS* (2nd ed.). New Delhi: All India Institute of Medical Sciences. Retrieved from https://www.aiims.edu/aiims/academic/aiims-syllabus/Syllabus%20-%20MBBS.pdf

Allen, H. (2007). *The Materia Medica of Nosodes.* B Jain Publishers.

Allen, T. (2021). *The Encyclopedia of Pure Materia Medica.* B Jain Publishers Private Limited. Retrieved from http://homeoint.org/allen/b/bell.htm

Alpert, J. (2006). Practicing Medicine in Plato's Cave. *The American Journal of Medicine, 119*, pp. 455-456. doi:10.1016/j.amjmed.2006.03.002

AMA. (2022). *Global Climate Change and Human Health H-135.938.* Retrieved from AMA Policy Finder: https://policysearch.ama-assn.org/policyfinder/detail/climate%20change?uri=%2FAMADoc%2FHOD.xml-0-309.xml

Aronson, L. (2019). *Elderhood: Redefining Aging, Transforming Medicine, Reimagining Life.* Bloomsbury Publishing.

Autier, P., & Boniol, M. (2018). Mammography screening: A major issue in medicine. *European Journal of Cancer, 90*, 34-62. doi:10.1016/j.ejca.2017.11.002

Baghi, A. (2000). *Rabindranath Tagore and His Medical World.* New Delhi: Konark Publishers.

Baker, M. (2016). 1,500 scientists lift the lid on reproducibility. *Nature, 533*, 452-454. doi:https://doi.org/10.1038/533452a

Bakken, J. S., Borody, T., Brandt, L. J., Brill, J. V., Demarco, D. C., Franzos, M. A., . . . Surawicz, C. (2011). Treating Clostridium difficile infection with fecal microbiota transplantation. *Clinical gastroenterology and hepatology, 9*(12), 1044-1049. doi:10.1016/j.cgh.2011.08.014

Barton, J., & Emanuel, E. (2005). The Patents-Based Pharmaceutical Development Process: Rationale, Problems, and Potential Reforms. *JAMA, 294*(16), 2075-2082. doi:10.1001/jama.294.16.2075

Basheer, S. (2012, December). The Invention of an Investment Incentive for Pharmaceutical Innovation. *The Journal of World Intellectual Property, 15*(5), 305-364. doi:10.1111/jwip.12001

Behring, A. (1905). *Moderne Phthisiogenetische und Phthisotherapeutische: Probleme in Historischer Beleuchtung.* Marburg.

Bellavite, P., Ortolani, R., Pontarollo, F., Pitari, G., & Conforti, A. (2007, June). mmunology and homeopathy: 5. The rationale of the 'Simile'. *Evidence-based complementary and alternative medicine: eCAM*, 149-163. doi:10.1093/ecam/nel117

Belon, P., Cumps, J., Mannajoni, P., Ste-Laudy, J., Roberfroid, M., & W. F. (1999). Inhibition of human basophil degranulation by successive histamine dilutions: results of a European multi-centre trial. *Infalammation Research, 48*, pp. 17-18.

Berridge, E. (1881). *The scientific use of Nosodes.* Retrieved from https://www.ncbi.nlm.nih.gov/pmc/articles/PMC9651766/pdf/homoeopathphys136631-0008.pdf

Bion, J., & Strunin, L. (1996). Multiple organ failure: from basic science to prevention (editorial). *British Journal of Anaesthesia, 77*(1-2), 1. doi:10.1093/bja/77.1.1

Blundon, E., Gallagher, R., & Ward, L. (2020, June 25). Electrophysiological evidence of preserved hearing at the end of life. *Nature: Scientific Reports, 10*(10336). doi:10.1038/s41598-020-67234-9

Borzelleca, J. (2000, January 1). Paracelsus: Herald of Modern Toxicology. *Toxicological Sciences, 53*(1). doi:https://doi.org/10.1093/toxsci/53.1.2

Braunwald, E., Hauser, S., Fauci, A., Longo, D., Kasper, D., & Jameson, J. (2000). *What is expected of the physician. The practice of medicine* (15th ed.). New York: McGraw-Hill.

Brennan, Z. (2020). Fauci: Hydroxychloroquine not effective against coronavirus. *Politico.*

Brien, S., Leydon, G., & Lewith, G. (2012). Homeopathy enables rheumatoid arthritis patients to cope with their chronic ill health: A qualitative study of patient's perceptions of the homeopathic consultation. *Patient Education and Counseling, 89*(3), pp. 507-516. doi:10.1016/j.pec.2011.11.008

Cagnacci, A., & Venier, M. (2019). The Controversial History of Hormone Replacement Therapy. *Medicina (Kaunas), 55*(9).

Cannon, W. (1929, July 1). Organization for Physiological Homeostasis. *Physiological Reviews*, July. doi:10.1152/physrev.1929.9.3.399

Carter, H., Winch, S., & Barnett, A. (2017, October 16). Incidence, duration and cost of futile treatment in end-of-life hospital admissions to three Australian public-sector tertiary hospitals: a retrospective multicentre cohort study. *BMJ Open*. doi:10.1136/bmjopen-2017-017661

Cartwright, T., & Torr, R. (2005). Making sense of illness: the experiences of users of complementary medicine. *Journal of Health Psychology, 10*(4), pp. 559-572. doi:10.1177/1359105305053425

Charon, R. (2008). Where does narrative medicine come from? In *Drives, diseases, attention and the body* (pp. 23-36). Albany, New York, USA: State University of New York Press.

Cherniack, E. (2010, April). Would the elderly be better off if they were given more placebos? *Geriatrics & Gerontology International, 10*(2), 131-137. doi:10.1111/j.1447-0594.2009.00580.x

Chikramane, P. S., Suresh, A. K., Bellare, J. R., & Kane, S. (2010, October). Extreme homeopathic dilutions retain starting materials: A nanoparticulate perspective. *Homeopathy*, pp. 231-242. doi:10.1016/j.homp.2010.05.006

Chirumbolo, S. (2011). Molecules and nanoparticles in extreme homeopathic dilutions: is Avogadro's Constant a dogma? *Homeopathy, 100*(3). doi:10.1016/j.homp.2011.02.015

Choudhary, A. (2022, August 23). *Profit driven corporatisation of healthcare system denies poor access to treatment: Chief Justice NV Ramana*. Retrieved from timesofindia.indiatimes: https://timesofindia.indiatimes.com/india/profit-driven-corporatisation-of-healthcare-system-denies-poor-access-to-treatment-chief-justice-nv-ramana/articleshow/93737531.cms

Cobb, L., Thomas, G., Dillard, D., Merndino, K., & Bruce, R. (1959, May 28). An Evaluation of Internal-Mammary-Artery Ligation by a Double-Blind Technic. *New England Journal of Medicine*, 1115-1118. doi:10.1056/NEJM195905282602204

Collins, F. (2019, December 17). *Aging research: Blood proteins show your age.* Retrieved from National Institute on Aging: https://www.nia.nih.gov/news/aging-research-blood-proteins-show-your-age#:~:text=The%20results%20offer%20important%20new,34%2C%2060%2C%20and%2078.

consumerfinance.gov. (2023, May 4). *Prepared Remarks of Director Rohit Chopra at the American Association of Healthcare Administration Management.* Retrieved from Consumer Financial Protection Bureau: https://www.consumerfinance.gov/about-us/newsroom/prepared-remarks-director-rohit-chopra-american-association-healthcare-administration-management/#3

Cyranoski, D. (2015, May 21). Artificial-windpipe surgeon committed misconduct. *Nature, 521*, 406-407. doi:10.1038/nature.2015.17605

da Costa, J. P., Vitorino, R., Silva, G., Vogel, C., Duarte, A. C., & Rocha-Santos, T. (2016). A synopsis on aging - Theories, mechanisms and future prospects. *Ageing Research Reviews, 29*, 90-112. doi:10.1016/j.arr.2016.06.005

Daniel, M. (2016, May 3). *News and Publications.* Retrieved from Johns Hopkins Medicine: https://www.hopkinsmedicine.org/news/media/releases/study_suggests_medical_errors_now_third_leading_cause_of_death_in_the_us

Dantas, F., & Rampes, H. (2000, July). Do homeopathic medicines provoke adverse effects? A systematic review. *British Homeopathic Journal.* doi:doi: 10.1054/homp.1999.0378

Dantas, F., Fisher, P., Walach, H., Wieland, F., Rastogi, D., Teixeira, H., . . . Weckx, L. (2007, January). A systematic review of the quality of homeopathic pathogenetic trials published from 1945 to 1995. *Homeopathy, 96*(1). doi:10.1016/j.homp.2006.11.005

Declercq, E., Young, R., Cabral, H., & Ecker, J. (2011, June). Is a rising cesarean delivery rate inevitable? Trends in industrialized countries, 1987 to 2007. *Birth, 38*(2), 99-104. doi:10.1111/j.1523-536X.2010.00459.x

Detsky, A., Gauthier,SR, & Fuchs, V. (2012, February). Specialization in medicine: how much is appropriate? *JAMA*, 463-464. doi:doi: 10.1001/jama.2012.44

Dewey, W. (1921). Homeopathy in influenza- A chorus of fifty in harmony. *Journal of the American Institute of Homeopathy*, 1038-1043.

Dhand, S. (2023, December 16). I'm a Physician: Why I want a Nurse Practitioner or PA as MY Doctor. Retrieved from https://youtu.be/O8wMvKS_aKU?si=XztRjPv0GKF3h3_m

Dhiman, R., Prakash, S. C., Sreenivas, V., & Puliyel, J. (2018). Correlation between Non-Polio Acute Flaccid Paralysis Rates with Pulse Polio Frequency in India. *International journal of environmental research and public health, 15*(8). doi:10.3390/ijerph15081755

Dmitry, B. (2017, May 1). *Mainstream Media Banned From Reporting On German Court's MMR Vaccine Ruling.* Retrieved from The People's Voice: https://thepeoplesvoice.tv/media-banned-german-court-mmr-vaccine-ruling/

Drugs,com. (n.d.). *Comparing Acetaminophen vs Tylenol.* Retrieved from drugs.com: https://www.drugs.com/compare/acetaminophen-vs-tylenol

Duffy, T. (2011, September). The Flexner Report — 100 Years Later. *The Yale Journal of Biology and Medicine, 84*(3), 269-276. Retrieved from https://www.ncbi.nlm.nih.gov/pmc/articles/PMC3178858/#:~:text=The%20Flexner%20Report%20of%201910,gold%20[st]andard%20of%20medical%20training.

Dutta, S. (2023, November 30). *Patterns of hysterectomy in India a 'concern', 66.8% done in pvt sector — report by OBGYN group, think tank.* Retrieved from theprint.in: https://theprint.in/health/95-hysterectomies-in-india-unnecessary-66-8-in-pvt-sector-report-by-obgyn-group-think-tank/1865540/

Džakula, A., Vočanec, D., & Lončarek, K. (2023). Fragmentation, dehumanization, commodification: crisis of medicine. *Croatian Medical Journal, 64*, 208-210. doi:10.3325/cmj.2023.64.208

Edmands, M., Hoff, L., Kaylor, L., Mower, L., & Sorrell, S. (2013, October 1). Bridging Gaps Between Mind, Body, & Spirit: Healing the Whole Person. *Journal of Psychosocial Nursing and Mental Health Services, 37*(10), 35-42. doi:10.3928/0279-3695-19991001-16

Elements of Health. (2023, July 4). *Homeopathy for the End of Life*. Retrieved from https://www.elementsofhealth.com.au/

Engel, G. (1977, April 8). The need for a new medical model: a challenge for biomedicine. *Science*, 129-136. doi:10.1126/science.847460

Enserink, M. (2010, December 24). French Nobelist Escapes 'Intellectual Terror' to Pursue Radical Ideas in China. *Science, 330*(6012), 1732. doi:10.1126/science.330.6012.1732

Epstein, R. (2020, June 8). *The Lancet's COVID Fiasco*. Retrieved from Hoover Institution: https://www.hoover.org/research/lancets-covid-fiasco

Fact.MR. (2023). *Homeopathic Products Market Outlook 2023 to 2033*. Retrieved from https://www.factmr.com/report/604/homeopathy-products-market

Fanelli, D. (2009, May 29). How many scientists fabricate and falsify research? A systematic review and meta-analysis of survey data. *PloS One*. doi:https://doi.org/10.1371/journal.pone.0005738

Frei, H. (2013). *Polarity Analysis in Homeopathy - A Precise Path to the Simillimum*. Kandern, Germany: Narayana Publishers.

Galtier, N., & Dutheil, J. (2007). Coevolution within and between genes. *Genome dynamics*, 1-12. doi:10.1159/ 000107599

Gerhard, D. (2024, February 15). A Science Sleuth Accuses a Harvard Medical School Neuroscientist of Research Misconduct. *The Scientist*. Retrieved from https://www.the-scientist.com/a-science-sleuth-accuses-a-harvard-medical-school-neuroscientist-of-research-misconduct-71652

Goldacre, B. (2013). *Bad Pharma: How Drug Companies Mislead Doctors and Harm Patients*. Farrar, Straus and Giroux.

Golden, I., & Bracho, G. (2014, July). A Reevaluation of the Effectiveness of Homoeoprophylaxis Against Leptospirosis in Cuba in 2007 and 2008. *Journal of Evidence Based Complementary Alternative Medicine*, 155-160. doi:doi: 10.1177/2156587214525402

Gorman, J. (2003, April 1). Aliens Inside Us: A (Mostly Friendly) Bacterial Nation. *New York Times*. Retrieved from https://www3.nd.edu/~hahn/pdf

Graham, D., Lundy, R., Benjamin, L., Kabler, J., Lewis, W., Kunish, N., & Graham, F. (1962). Specific Attitudes in Initial Interviews with Patients Having Specific "Psychosomatic" Diseases. *Psychosomatic Medicine, XXIV*(2), 257-266.

Graham, D., Stern, J., & Winokur, G. (1958). Experimental Investigation of the Specificity of Attitude Hypothesis in Psychosomatic Disease. *Psychosomatic Medicine, XX*(6), 446-457.

Guinane, C., & Cotter, P. (2013). Role of the gut microbiota in health and chronic gastrointestinal disease: understanding a hidden metabolic organ. *Therapeutic advances in gastroenterology, 6*(4), 295-308. doi:10.1177/ 1756283X13482996

Gupta, N., Singh, R., & Saxena, R. (2019). Clinical Evaluation of Homoeopathic Medicines in Benign Prostatic Hyperplasia. *Homœopathic Links*. doi:10.1055/ s-0039-1693154

Hagan, J. (2015). Medicine at Death's Door: One Chance to Get It Right. *Missouri Medicine, 112*(3), 148-150.

Hahnemann, S. (2013). *Organon of the Medical Art*. Palo Alto, CA, USA: Birdcage Books.

Hansen, A. (2018, May 10). Brand name or generic? Study probes use of drug names, which ties to health care costs. *Scope*.

Harvard Medical School. (2021, December 13). *Harvard Health Publishing - Mental Health*. Retrieved from https://www.health.harvard.edu/mental-health/ the-power-of-the-placebo-effect

Hazan, S., Stollman, N., Bozkurt, H., Dave, S., Papoutsis, A., Daniels, J., . . . Borody, T. (2022). Lost microbes of COVID-19: Bifidobacterium, Faecalibacterium depletion and decreased microbiome diversity associated with SARS-CoV-2 infection severity. *BMJ Open Gastroenterology, 9*. doi:10.1136/ bmjgast-2022-000871

Helman, C. (1981, September). Diseaseversus illness ingeneral practice. *Journal o fth eRoyal College of GeneralPractitioners*, 548-552. Retrieved from www.ncbi. nlm.nih.gov/pmc/articles/PMC1972172/pdf/jroyalcgprac00105-0038.pdf

Horton, R. (2014, March 11). The Dawn of McScience. *New York Review of Books, 51*(4), 7-9.

House of Commons. (2010). *Science and Technology Committee.* Report, together with formal minutes, oral and written evidence. Retrieved from https://publications.parliament.uk/pa/cm200910/cmselect/cmsctech/45/45.pdf

Hróbjartsson, A., & & Gøtzsche, P. (2010). Placebo interventions for all clinical conditions. *The Cochrane database of systematic reviews.* doi:10.1002/14651858. CD003974.pub3

Humphries, S., & Bystrianyk, R. (2013). *Dissolving Illusions: Disease, Vaccines, and the Forgotten History.* CreateSpace Independent Publishing Platform.

Hunsaker, A. (1999, August). Pathography: patient narratives of illness. *Wall Street Journal, 171,* 127-129. Retrieved from https://edisciplinas.usp.br/pluginfile.php/7668526/mod_resource/content/1/1999%20Hawkings%20Pathographies.pdf

Hunter, K. (1991). *Doctors' stories: the narrative structure of medical knowledge.* Princeton NJ: Princeton University Press.

Igho, J., Carl, J., & Aronson, J. (2016). Worldwide withdrawal of medicinal products because of adverse drug reactions: a systematic review and analysis. *Critical Reviews in Toxicology, 46*(6), 477-489. doi:10.3109/10408444.2016.1149452

Illich, I. (1974). Medical nemesis. *The BMJ.* doi:http://dx.doi.org/10.1136/jech.57.12.919

Ioannidis, J. (2014, October 21). How to Make More Published Research True. *PLoS Med, 11*(10). doi:https://doi.org/ 10.1371/journal

Ioannidis, J., Klavans, R., & Boyack, K. (2018, September 12). Thousands of scientists publish a paper every five days. *Nature.* Retrieved from https://www.nature.com/articles/d41586-018-06185-8

Iyer, M. (2015, January 4). *44% advised unnecessary surgery: 2nd opinion-givers.* Retrieved from times of India.indiatimes: https://timesofindia.indiatimes.com/india/ 44-advised-unnecessary-surgery-2nd-opinion-givers/articleshow/ 45746903.cms

Jadad, A., & Enkin, M. (2007). *Randomized Controlled Trials: Questions, Answers and Musings* (2nd ed.). BMJ Books/Blackwell Publishing.

Jäger, T., Würtenberger, S., & Baumgartner, S. (2021, May). Effects of Homeopathic Preparations of Mercurius corrosivus on the Growth Rate of Moderately

Mercury-Stressed Duckweed Lemna gibba L. *Homeopathy: the journal of the Faculty of Homeopathy, 110*(2), pp. 122-131. doi:10.1055/s-0040-1718743

Johns Hopkins Medicine. (2016, May 3). *Study Suggests Medical Errors Now Third Leading Cause of Death in the U.S.* Retrieved from News and Publications: https://www.hopkinsmedicine.org/news/media/releases/study_suggests_medical_errors_now_third_leading_cause_of_death_in_the_us

Jones, D. (2013). Visions of a Cure: Visualization, Clinical Trials, and Controversies in Cardiac Therapeutics. In S. G. Kaiser, *Science and the American Century: Readings from "Isis".* The University of Chicago Press.

Jox, R., Schaider, A., Marckmann, G., & Borasio, G. (2012). Medical futility at the end of life: the perspectives of intensive care and palliative care clinicians. *Journal of Medical Ethics, 38*, 540-545. doi:10.1136/medethics-2011-100479

Jutte, R. (2014). Hahnemann and placebo. *Homeopathy, 103*, pp. 208-212. doi:10.1016/j.homp.2014.03.003

Kabat, G. (2017). *Taking distrust of science seriously.* EMBO Reports. doi:10.15252/embr.201744294

Karp, J., Sanchez, C., Guilbert, P., Mina, W., Demonceaux, A., & Curé, H. (2016). Treatment with Ruta graveolens 5CH and Rhus toxicodendron 9CH may reduce joint pain and stiffness linked to aromatase inhibitors in women with early breast cancer: results of a pilot observational study. *Homeopathy*, 299-308. doi:10.1016/j.homp.2016.05.004

Kasprak, A. (2020). *Has Dr. Zelenko Successfully Treated 669 Coronavirus Patients?* Retrieved from Snopes Fact Check: https://www.snopes.com/fact-check/zelenko-669-coronavirus-patients/

Kaur, H., Chalia, D. S., & Manchanda, R. K. (2019, May). Homeopathy in Public Health in India. *Homeopathy, 108*(2), 76-87. doi:10.1055/s-0038-1673710

Kent, J. (2008). *Lectures on Homeopathic Philosophy.* New Delhi: B Jain Publishers.

Kent, J. (2011). *Lectures on Homeopathic Materia Medica.* New Delhi: B Jain Publishers Pvt Ltd.

Khanna, K., & Chandra, S. (1976, September). Control of tomato fruit rot caused by Fusarium roseus with homoeopathic drugs. *Indian Phytopathology*, pp. 269-272.

Khuda-Bukhsh, A., Mondal, J., & Shah, R. (2017). Therapeutic potential of HIV nosode 30c as evaluated in A549 lung cancer cells. *Homeopathy, 106*(4), 203-213. doi:doi: 10.1016/j.homp.2017.09.001

Kleijnen,. J., Knipschild, P., & Riet, t. (1991, February 9). Clinical trials of homeopathy. *British Medical Journal*, 316-323.

Kleinman, A. (2020). *The Illness Narratives - Suffering, Healing, And The Human Condition.* Basic Books.

Klienman, A. (1995). What is specific to Biomedicine? In *Writings at the margin: Discourse between Anthropology and Medicine* (pp. 21-40). Berkeley: University of California Press.

Knappen, L. (2013). Being evidence based in the absence of evidence: The management of non-evidence in guideline development. *Social Studies of Science, 43*(5), 681-706.

Konitzer, M., Renee, A., & Doering, T. (2003, April). Homeopathic remedies as metaphors in family therapy. A narrative-based approach to homeopathy. *Homeopathy, 92*(2), 77-83. doi:10.1016/S1475-4916(03)00005-5

Konnitzer, M. (2005). Narrative based medicine. Re-introduction of the subject in medicine? *Sozialer Sinn.*, 111-129.

Kumar, R. (2023, August). The curious case of extinction of family physicians from the Indian Health System – An open letter to the members of the National Medical Commission: Draft competency-based medical education curriculum regulations 2023 – Complete exclusion of family physi. *Journal of Family Medicine and Primary Care, 12*(8). doi:10.4103/jfmpc.jfmpc_1323_23

Lancet. (2010, May 15). Uncertainty in medicine. *The Lancet.* doi:10.1016/S0140-6736(10)60719-2

Lancet. (2020, May 16). Reviving the US CDC. *The Lancet, 395*(10236), 1521. doi:https://doi.org/10.1016/S0140-6736(20)31140-5

Lecroy, K. (2001). *American Family Physician Journal.* Retrieved from https://www.aafp.org/pubs/afp/issues/2001/1215/p1942.html

Levenson, R. (2019). Stress and Illness: A Role for Specific Emotions. *Psychosomatic Medicine, 81*(8), 720-730. doi:10.1097/PSY.0000000000000736

Lo, A., & Mueller, M. (2010). Warning: Physics Envy May be Hazardous to Your Wealth! *Journal of Investment Management*. doi:Lo, Andrew W. and Mueller, Mark T., Warning: Physics Envy May be Hazardous to Your Wealth! (March 12,10.2139/ssrn.1563882

Lorenzetti, E., Stangarlin, J., & Kuhn, O. (2017). Antimicrobial activity against Macrophomina phaseolina and the control of charcoal rot in soybeans using the homoeopathic drugs Sepia and Arsenicum album. *Archives of Institutional Biology, 84*. doi:10.1590/1808-1657000562016

Lose, G., & Klarskov, N. (2017, July 13). Why published research is untrustworthy. *International Urogynecology Journal*(28), pp. 1271-1274. doi:0.1007/s00192-017-3389-1

Macleod, M., Michie, S., Roberts, I., Dirnagl, U., Chalmers, I., Ioannidis, J., . . . Glasziou, P. (2014, January 11). Biomedical research: increasing value, reducing waste. *Lancet, 383*(9912). doi:doi: 10.1016/S0140-6736(13)62329-6

Mathie, R. (2003). The research evidence base for homeopathy: a fresh assessment of the literature. *Homeopathy, 92*(2), 84-91. doi:10.1016/S1475-4916(03)00006-7

MayoClinic. (2023). *Coronavirus disease 2019 (COVID-19)*. Retrieved November 3, 2023, from Mayo Clinic: https://www.mayoclinic.org/diseases-conditions/coronavirus/diagnosis-treatment/drc-20479976#:~:text=No%20cure%20is%20available%20for,and%20older%20in%20the%20hospital.

Mehra, M. R., Desai, S., & Patel, A. (2020). Hydroxychloroquine or chloroquine with or without a macrolide for treatment of COVID-19: a multinational registry analysis. *The Lancet*. doi:https://doi.org/10.1016/S0140-6736(20)31180-6

Meissner, K. (2011, June 27). The placebo effect and the autonomic nervous system: evidence for an intimate relationship. *Philosophical transactions of the Royal Society of London. Series B, Biological sciences, 366*(1572), 1808-1817. doi:10.1098/rstb.2010.0403

Milgrom, L. (2003). Patient–practitioner–remedy (PPR) entanglement. Part3. Refining the quantum metaphor for homeopathy. *Homeopathy, 92*, 152-160. doi:10.1016/S1475-4916(03)00038-9

Millard, E. (2023, May 24). How Nutrition Education for Doctors Is Evolving. *Time 2030*. Retrieved from https://time.com/6282404/nutrition-education-doctors/

Mirilli, J. (2009, March 15). Thematic Repertory and Materia Medica of the Mind Symptoms. *Homeopathy for Everyone*. Retrieved from https://hpathy.com/homeopathy-repertory/thematic-repertory-and-materia-medica-of-the-mind-symptoms/

Mittal, R., Khurana, A., Ghosh, M., Bawaskar, R., Taneja, D., Kashyap, S., & Manchanda, R. (2016, July). An open-label pilot study to explore usefulness of Homoeopathic treatment in nonerosive gastroesophageal reflux disease. *Indian Journal of Research in Homoeopathy, 10*(3), 188-198. doi:10.4103/0974-7168.188240

Mondal, J., Das, J., Shah, R., & Khudabukhsh, A. (2016, May). A homeopathic nosode, Hepatitis C 30 demonstrates anticancer effect against liver cancer cells in vitro by modulating telomerase and topoisomerase II activities as also by promoting apoptosis via intrinsic mitochondrial pathway. *Journal of Integrative Medicine, 14*(3), 209-218. doi:https://doi.org/10.1016/S2095-4964(16)60251-0

Mondal, J., Samadder, A., & Khudabukhsh, A. (2016). *Journal of Integrative Medicine, 14*(2), 143-153. doi:https://doi.org/10.1016/S2095-4964(16)60230-3

Morrow, A. (2023, March 15). *End-of-Life Stages Timeline: What to expect as someone nears death*. Retrieved from verywell health: https://www.verywellhealth.com/the-journey-towards-death-1132504

Motiwala, F., Kundu, T., Bagmar, K., Kakatkar, V., & Dhole, Y. (2016, July). Effect of Homoeopathic treatment on Activity of Daily Living (ADL) in Knee Osteoarthritis: A prospective observational study. *Indian Journal of Research in Homoeopathy, 10*(3), 182-187. doi:10.4103/0974-7168.188238

Moynihan, R., Heath, I., & Henry, D. (2002). Selling sickness: the pharmaceutical industry and disease mongering. *BMJ - Clinical Research Edition, 324*(7342), 886-891. doi:10.1136/bmj.324.7342.886

Nair, K., Gopinadhan, S., & Kurup, T. (2014). Homoeopathic Genus Epidemicus 'Bryonia alba' as a prophylactic during an outbreak of Chikungunya in

India: A cluster -randomised, double -blind, placebo- controlled trial. *Indian Journal of Research in Homoeopathy, 8*(3). Retrieved from https://www.ijrh. org/journal/vol8/iss3/6/

Nayak, D., & Varanasi, R. (2020). Homoeopathic nosodes, a neglected approach for epidemics: A critical review. *Indian J Res Homoeopathy*, 129-135. doi:10.4103/ijrh.ijrh_46_20

Negro, F., & Marino, F. (2021, November 7). Homeopathy in Epidemics: From Cholera to 1918 Spanish Flu (Part 2). *OBM Integrative and Complementary Medicine, 6*(4). doi:doi:10.21926/obm.icm.2104045

NHMRC. (2015). *Administrative Report: NHMRC Advice on the effectiveness of homeopathy for treating health conditions.* Canberra: NHMRC. Retrieved from www.nhmrc.gov.au/guidelines-publications/cam02

NHS. (2021, April 7). *Homeopathy.* Retrieved from nhs.uk: https://www.nhs.uk/ conditions/homeopathy/

Nuffield Trust. (2020). *Privatisation in the English NHS: Implications of Covid-19.* London: London School of Economics. Retrieved from https://www.lse. ac.uk/health-policy/assets/documents/EHPG-180920/EHPG-Sarah-Reed-NHS-Privatisation.pdf

Oberbaum, M., Schreiber, R., Rosenthal, C., & Itzchaki, M. (2003, January). Homeopathic treatment in emergency medicine: a case series. *Homeopathy*, 44-47. doi:10.1054/homp.2002.0071

Ouyang, D., Tisdale, R., Ashley, E., Chi, J., & Chen, J. (2018). Acetaminophen or Tylenol? A Retrospective Analysis of Medication Digital Communication Practices. *ournal of general internal medicine, 33*(8), 1218-1220. doi:10.1007/ s11606-018-4455-1

Panek, R. (2019). *The Trouble with Gravity: Solving the Mystery Beneath Our Feet.* United States: Harper Collins.

Paterson, J. (2017). *The Bowel Nosodes.* Kalpaz Publications.

Paulus, V., & Ravi, A. (2024, February 1). Top Harvard Medical School Neuroscientist Accused of Research Misconduct. *The Harvard Crimson.* Retrieved from https://www.thecrimson.com/article/2024/2/1/harvard-neuroscientist-research-misconduct/

Pead, P. (2006, December 23). Benjamin Jesty: the first vaccinator revealed. *The Lancet, 368*(9554). doi:https://doi.org/10.1016/S0140-6736(06)69878-4

Pérez-Jover, V., Mira, J. J., Carratala-Munuera, C., Gil-Guillen, V. F., Basora, J., López-Pineda, A., & Orozco-Beltrán, D. (2018, February 10). Inappropriate Use of Medication by Elderly, Polymedicated, or Multipathological Patients with Chronic Diseases. *International Journal of Environmental Research and Public Health, 15*(2). doi:10.3390/ijerph15020310

Pillai, A., Koduri, K., Gokhale, Y., & Venkatesh, M. (2021, June). Auditing the efficacy of prophylactic measures against Covid-19 amongst Healthcare workers in India. *J Infect, 82*(6), 16-17. doi:10.1016/j.jinf.2021.03.022

Prajapati, S., Mahima, S., & Kumar, A. (2019). Antimicrobial activity of different homoeopathic drugs and their potencies against 'Aspergillus niger' In vitro. *Indian Journal of Research in Homoeopathy, 13*(3), pp. 150-158. doi:10.4103/ijrh.ijrh_46_18

Prasad, R. (2007, November 17). Homoeopathy booming in India. *The Lancet, 370*(9600), 1679-1680. doi:10.1016/S0140-6736(07)61709-7

Rahe, R. (1968). Life-change measurement as a predictor of illness. *Proceedings of the Royal Society of Medicine, 61*(11), 1124-1126.

RajGuru, A. (2015, September 17). Dr. Amarsinh D Nikam MD(Hom) Interviewed by Ashok RajGuru. *Hpathy*. Retrieved from https://hpathy.com/homeopathy-interviews/dr-amarsinh-d-nikam-mdhom-interviewed-by-ashok-rajguru/

RajGuru, A. (2021, April 17). In Conversation with Dr. Rajesh Shah – The Developer of a COVID-19 Nosode. *Hpathy*. Retrieved from https://hpathy.com/homeopathy-interviews/in-conversation-with-dr-rajesh-shah-the-developer-of-a-covid-19-nosode/

Ramakrishnan, A., & Coulter, C. (2001). *A Homeopathic Approach to Cancer.* Berkeley Spring, WV: Ninth House Publishing.

Rambhade, S., Chakarborty, Shrivastava, A., Patil, U. K., & Rambhade, A. (2012). A survey on polypharmacy and use of inappropriate medications. *Toxicology international, 19*(1), 68-73. doi:10.4103/0971-6580.94506

Rao, M., & Pilot, E. (2014). The missing link--the role of primary care in global health. *Global Health Action, 7.* doi:10.3402/gha.v7.23693

Regis, E. (2020, February 1). No One Can Explain Why Planes Stay in the Air. *Scientific American*. Retrieved from https://www.scientificamerican.com/article/no-one-can-explain-why-planes-stay-in-the-air/#:~:text=The%20theory%20states%20that%20a,back%20upward%2C%20which%20is%20lift.

Rehman, A. (2004). *Encyclopedia of Remedy Relationship in Homeopathy*. Stuttgart: Medizinischer Verlag.

Reilly, D., Taylor, M., Beattie, N., Campbell, J., McSharry, C., Aitchison, T., . . . Stevenson, R. (1994). Is evidence for homoeopathy reproducible? *The Lancet, 344*(8637). doi:10.1016/s0140-6736(94)90407-3

Remignanti, D. (2024, February 20). *The Doctor Will Not See You Now*. Retrieved from BMJ Blogs - Medical Humanities: https://blogs.bmj.com/medical-humanities/2024/02/20/the-doctor-will-not-see-you-now/#:~:text=can%20be%20daunting.-,Dr.,is%20something%20a%20man%20has.%E2%80%9D

Ritter, J., Lewis, L., Mant, T., & Ferro, A. (2008). *A Tetbook of Clinical Pharmacology and Therapeutics* (5th ed.). Boca Raton: CRC Press, Taylor & Francis Group.

Roduner, E. (2006). Size matters: why nanomaterials are different. *Chemical Society Reviews, 35*(7), pp. 583-592. doi:10.1039/b502142c

Rostock, M., Naumann, J., Guethlin, C., Guenther, L., Bartsch, H., & Walach, H. (2011, January 17). Classical homeopathy in the treatment of cancer patients--a prospective observational study of two independent cohorts. *BMC Cancer*. doi:10.1186/1471-2407-11-19

Rothwell, P. (2005). External validity of randomized controlled trials: "To whom do the results of this trial apply?". *The Lancet*(365), 82-89.

Roughead, E., & Semple, S. (2009). *Medication safety in acute care in Australia: Where are we now? Part 1: a review of the extent and causes of medication problems 2002–2008*. Australia and New Zealand Health Policy 2009.

Saha, S. (2010). Syphilinum: An Answerto Osteoporosis. *Homeopathic Links*, 155-159.

Sanchez-Pramo, C., Hill, R., Mahler, D., Narayan, A., & Yonzan, N. (2021, October 7). *COVID-19 leaves a legacy of rising poverty and widening inequality*. Retrieved from World Bank Blogs: https://blogs.worldbank.org/

developmenttalk/covid-19-leaves-legacy-rising-poverty-and-widening-inequality#:~:text=The%20result%20is%20that%20the,percent%20are%20down%202.8%20percent.

Saxena, A., Pandey, M., & Gupta, R. (1987). Effect of certain homeopathic drugs on incidence of seed-borne fungi and seed germination of Abelmoschus esculentus. *Indian Journal of Mycology & Plant Pathology, 17*, pp. 191-192.

Schuster, P. (2011, July). Is there a Newton of the blade of grass? The Complex Relation Between Mathematics, Physics, and Biology. *Complexity, 16*(6), 5-9. doi:10.1002/cplx.20381

Science. (2010, December 24). French Nobelist Escapes 'IntellectualTerror' to Pursue Radical Ideas in China. *Science*, pp. 1732-1734.

Seegert, L. (2019, June 27). *Doctors are ageist — and it's harming older patients.* Retrieved from THINK - Opinion, Analysis, Essays: https://www.nbcnews.com/think/opinion/doctors-are-ageist-it-s-harming-older-patients-ncna1022286

Serra-Garcia, M., & Gneezy, U. (2021, May 21). Nonreplicable publications are cited more than replicable ones. *Science Advances*. doi:doi: 10.1126/sciadv.abd1705

Shah, R. (2011, September). What Homeopathy is Not. *Homeopathic Links, 24*, pp. 142-144.

Shah, R. (2020). Preparation of Coronavirus Nosodes Sourced from a Clinical Sample of SARS-Cov-2 Positive Patient, Inactivated Strain, and Spike Glycoprotein. *International Journal of High Dilution Research, 19*(4), 2-9.

Shmerling, R. (2021, July 13). *Is our healthcare system broken?* Retrieved from Harvard Health Publishing/Blog: https://www.health.harvard.edu/blog/is-our-healthcare-system-broken-202107132542

Singh, Y., Eisenberg, M., & Sood, N. (2023, March). Factors Associated With Public Trust in Pharmaceutical Manufacturers. *JAMA Network Open, 6*(3). doi:doi: 10.1001/jamanetworkopen

SIPRI. (2022, December 5). *Arms sales of SIPRI Top 100 arms companies grow despite supply chain challenges.* Retrieved from pri.org/media/press-release/2022/arms-sales-sipri-top-100-arms-companies-grow-despite-supply-chain-challenges#:~:text=(Stockholm%2C%205%20December%20 2022),Peace%20Research%20Institute%20(SIPRI).

Smith, R. (2005). Medical Journals are an Extension of the Marketing Arm of Pharmaceutical Companies. *PLoS.*

Solomon, M. (2015). On narrative medicine. In M. Solomon, *Making medical knowledge* (pp. 178-205). Oxford: Oxford University Press.

Sourdet, S., Lafont, C., Rolland, Y., Nourhashemi, F., Andrieu, S., & Vellas, B. (2015, August 1). Preventable Iatrogenic Disability in Elderly Patients During Hospitalization. *J Am Med Dir Assoc.* doi:doi: 10.1016/j.jamda.2015.03.011

Stange, K. (2009, March). The Problem of Fragmentation and the Need for Integrative Solutions. *Annals of Family Medicine,* 100-103. doi:doi: 10.1370/ afm.971

Statista. (2023). *Revenue of the worldwide pharmaceutical market from 2001 to 2022.* Statista. Retrieved from https://www.statista.com/statistics/263102/ pharmaceutical-market-worldwide-revenue-since-2001/

Steel, K., Gertman, P., Crescenzi, C., & Anderson, J. (2004, February). Iatrogenic illness on a general medical service at a university hospital. *Qual Saf Health Care.* doi:10.1136/qshc.2002.003830

Takayama, M. (2021). Medical Hegemony and Healthcare: Centrality in Healthcare. In A. Agrawal, & S. Kosgi, *Healthcare Access.* doi:DOI: 10.5772/ intechopen.99174

Tanaka, Y. (2018, February 1). Case Study of Homeopathic Bowel Nosode Remedies for Dysbiotic Japanese Patients. *The Journal of Alternative & Complementary Medicine, 24*(2), 187-192. doi:10.1089/acm.2017.0061

Teut, M., Lüdtke, R., Schnabel, K., Willich, S., & Witt, C. (2010, February 22). Homeopathic treatment of elderly patients--a prospective observational study with follow-up over a two year period. *BMC Geriatrics.* doi:doi. org/10.1186/1471-2318-10-10

Thakur, B. (2016, January 7). *Homeopathy is bogus, harmful: Nobel laureate Venkatraman Ramakrishnan.* Retrieved from Hindustan Times: https://www.

hindustantimes.com/india/homeopathy-astrology-are-bogus-says-nobel-laureate-venkatraman-ramakrishna/story-oNNzWBnosMFiLnrnmfkdxI.html

The Nobel Prize Foundation. (2023). *The Nobel Prize in Physiology or Medicine 1927*. Retrieved from The Nobel Prize: https://www.nobelprize.org/prizes/medicine/1927/summary/

Thomas, Y. (2007). The history of the Memory of Water. *Homeopathy, 96*, pp. 151-157. doi:10.1016/j.homp.2007. 03.006

TOI. (2023, September 26). Farmers now study how homeopathy can help cure crops. *Times of India*. Retrieved from https://timesofindia.indiatimes.com/blogs/tracking-indian-communities/farmers-now-study-how-homeopathy-can-help-cure-crops/

Toledo, M., Stangarlin, J., & Bonato, C. (2011). Homeopathy for the control of plant pathogens. *Science against microbial pathogens: communicating current research and technological advances*. Retrieved from www.considera.org/downloads/Published%20Papers/homeopathy-for-the-control-of-plant-pathogens.pdf

Ullman, D. (2007). *The Homeopathic Revolution: Why Famous People and Cultural Heroes Love Homeopathy*. Berkeley: North Atlantic Books.

US Food & Drug Administration. (2020, July 4). *Fecal Microbiota for Transplantation: Safety Alert - Risk of Serious Adverse Events Likely Due to Transmission of Pathogenic Organisms*. Retrieved from fda.gov: https://www.fda.gov/safety/medical-product-safety-information/fecal-microbiota-transplantation-safety-alert-risk-serious-adverse-events-likely-due-transmission

Viksveen, P. R. (2017). Depressed patients' experiences with and perspectives on treatment provided by homeopaths. A qualitative interview study embedded in a trial. *European Journal of Integrative Medicine, 15*, pp. 73-80. doi:10.1016/j.eujim.2017.09.004

Viksveen, P., Fibert, P., & Relton, C. (2018, September). Homeopathy in the treatment of depression: a systematic review. *European Journal of Integrative Medicine, 22*, 22-36. doi:10.1016/j.eujim.2018.07.004

Vora, P. (2017, July 3). *Patients pay a heavy price as India's doctors continue with the corrupt 'cut practice'*. Retrieved from scroll.in/pulse: https://scroll.in/

pulse/842492/patients-pay-a-heavy-price-as-indias-doctors-continue-with-the-corrupt-cut-practice

Wager, T., & Atlas, L. (2015, July). The neuroscience of placebo effects: connecting context, learning and health. *Nature Reviews Neuroscience*, pp. 403-418. doi:10.1038/nrn3976

Wani, K. S., Prabhune, A., Jadhav, A., Ranjekar, P., & Kaul-Ghanekar, R. (2016). Evaluating the anticancer activity and nanoparticulate nature of homeopathic preparations of Terminalia chebula. *Homeopathy, 105*(4), pp. 318-326. doi:10.1016/j.homp.2016.02.004

Wartolowska, K., Judge, A., Hopewell, S., Collins, G., Dean, B., Rombach, . . . Carr, A. (2014, May). Use of placebo controls in the evaluation of surgery: systematic review. *BMJ (Clinical Research edition), 21*(348). doi:10.1136/bmj.g3253

Wassenhoven, M., & Ives, G. (2004). An observational study of patients receiving homeopathic treatment. *Homeopathy, 93*, 3-11. doi:10.1016/j.homp.2003.11.010

Whitmont, R. (2020). The Human Microbiome, Conventional Medicine, and Homeopathy. *Homeopathy, 109*(4), pp. 248-255. doi:10.1055/s-0040-1709665

WHO. (2018, March 14). *Poliomyelitis: Does polio still exist? Is it curable?* Retrieved from World Health Organization: https://www.who.int/news-room/questions-and-answers/item/does-polio-still-exist-is-it-curable

Wholihan, D. (2016). Seeing the Light: End-of-Life Experiences—Visions, Energy Surges, and Other Death Bed Phenomena. *Nursing Clinics of North America, 51*(3), 489-500. doi:10.1016/j.cnur.2016.05.005

Willmott, L., White, B., Gallois, C., Parker, M., Graves, N., Winch, S., . . . Close, E. (2016). Reasons doctors provide futile treatment at the end of life: a qualitative study. *Journal of Medical Ethics*, 496-503.

Wolf, Y., Katsnelson, M., & Koonin, E. (2018). Physical foundations of biological complexity. *Proceedings of the National Academy of Sciences, 115*(37), 8678-8687. doi:10.1073/pnas.1807890115

Yang, Z., Jiang, Y., Li, F. L., & Zhao, Z. (2023). Efficacy of SARS-CoV-2 vaccines and the dose–response relationship with three major antibodies: a systematic review and meta-analysis of randomised controlled trials. *The Lancet Microbe, 4*(4). doi:https://doi.org/10.1016/S2666-5247(22)00390-1

Zhang, Y., Li, S., Gan, R., Zhou, T., Xu, D., & Li, H. (2015, April 2). Impacts of gut bacteria on human health and diseases. *International journal of molecular sciences, 16*(4), 7493-7519. doi:10.3390/ijms16047493

Zhao, M., Chen, Z., Xu, T., Fan, P., & Tian, F. (2023, August 24). Global prevalence of polypharmacy and potentially inappropriate medication in older patients with dementia: a systematic review and meta-analysis. *Frontiers in Pharmacology, 14.*

Zhou, E. S., Hall, K. T., Michaud, A. L., Blackmon, J. E., Partridge, A. H., & Recklitis, C. J. (2019, June). Open-label placebo reduces fatigue in cancer survivors: a randomized trial. *Supportive care in cancer: official journal of the Multinational Association of Supportive Care in Cancer, 27*(6), 2179-2187. doi:10.1007/s00520-018-4477-6

Index